Basic and ~~Clinical Science Course~~

# Glaucoma
## Section 10

# 2002–2003
(Last major revision 2000–2001)

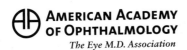

**AMERICAN ACADEMY
OF OPHTHALMOLOGY**
*The Eye M.D. Association*

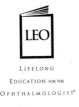

LEO

LIFELONG
EDUCATION FOR THE
OPHTHALMOLOGIST®

The Basic and Clinical Science Course is one component of the Lifelong Education for the Ophthalmologist (LEO) framework, which assists members in planning their continuing medical education. LEO includes an array of clinical education products that members may select to form individualized, self-directed learning plans for updating their clinical knowledge. Active members or fellows who use LEO components may accumulate sufficient CME credits to earn the LEO Award. Contact the Academy's Clinical Education Division for further information on LEO.

The American Academy of Ophthalmology is accredited by the Accreditation Council for Continuing Medical Education to provide continuing medical education for physicians.

The American Academy of Ophthalmology designates this educational activity for a maximum of 30 hours in category 1 credit toward the AMA Physician's Recognition Award. Each physician should claim only those hours of credit that he/she has actually spent in the activity.

The Academy provides this material for educational purposes only. It is not intended to represent the only or best method or procedure in every case, nor to replace a physician's own judgment or give specific advice for case management. Including all indications, contraindications, side effects, and alternative agents for each drug or treatment is beyond the scope of this material. All information and recommendations should be verified, prior to use, with current information included in the manufacturers' package inserts or other independent sources, and considered in light of the patient's condition and history. Reference to certain drugs, instruments, and other products in this publication is made for illustrative purposes only and is not intended to constitute an endorsement of such. Some material may include information on applications that are not considered community standard, that reflect indications not included in approved FDA labeling, or that are approved for use only in restricted research settings. The FDA has stated that it is the responsibility of the physician to determine the FDA status of each drug or device he or she wishes to use, and to use them with appropriate patient consent in compliance with applicable law. The Academy specifically disclaims any and all liability for injury or other damages of any kind, from negligence or otherwise, for any and all claims that may arise from the use of any recommendations or other information contained herein.

# Basic and Clinical Science Course

Thomas J. Liesegang, MD, Jacksonville, Florida
*Senior Secretary for Clinical Education*

Thomas A. Deutsch, MD, Chicago, Illinois
*Secretary for Instruction*

M. Gilbert Grand, MD, St. Louis, Missouri
*BCSC Course Chair*

# Section 10

## Faculty Responsible for This Edition

Louis Cantor, MD, *Chair,* Indianapolis, Indiana

Robert D. Fechtner, MD, Newark, New Jersey

Andrew J. Michael, MD, Richmond, Virginia

Steven T. Simmons, MD, Albany, New York

M. Roy Wilson, MD, Omaha, Nebraska

Steven V.L. Brown, MD, Evanston, Illinois
*Practicing Ophthalmologists Advisory Committee for Education*

The authors state the following financial relationships:

Dr. Brown: speaker/panel moderator for Allergan Inc; Merck & Co, Inc; Pharmacia & Upjohn Co.

Dr. Cantor: research funding from Alcon Laboratories Inc; Allergan Inc; CIBA; Merck & Co, Inc; Pharmacia & Upjohn Co; speakers bureau of Allergan Inc; Merck & Co, Inc.

Dr. Fechtner: research funding, consulting, or speakers bureau for Alcon Laboratories Inc; Allergan Inc; CIBA; Merck & Co, Inc; Pharmacia & Upjohn Co.

Dr. Simmons: research funding from Alcon Laboratories Inc; Allergan Inc; CIBA; Merck & Co, Inc; speakers bureau of Allergan Inc; CIBA; Merck & Co, Inc.

The other authors state that they have no significant financial interest or other relationship with the manufacturer of any commercial product discussed in the chapters that they contributed to this publication or with the manufacturer of any competing commercial product.

## Recent Past Faculty

A. Robert Bellows, MD

Michael S. Berlin, MD

Frank G. Berson, MD

Elizabeth A. Hodapp, MD

Michael A. Kass, MD

David A. Lee, MD

Stephen B. Lichtenstein, MD

Bradford J. Shingleton, MD

Robert L. Stamper, MD

Richard Stone, MD

In addition, the Academy gratefully acknowledges the contributions of numerous past faculty and advisory committee members who have played an important role in the development of previous editions of the Basic and Clinical Science Course.

**American Academy of Ophthalmology Staff**

Hal Straus
*Director, Publications Department*

Margaret Denny
*Managing Editor*

Jack Daniel
*Medical Editor*

Maxine Garrett
*Administrative Coordinator*

American Academy of Ophthalmology
655 Beach Street
Box 7424
San Francisco, CA 94120-7424

# CONTENTS

# GENERAL INTRODUCTION

The Basic and Clinical Science Course (BCSC) is designed to meet the needs of residents and practitioners for a comprehensive yet concise curriculum of the field of ophthalmology. The BCSC has developed from its original brief outline format, which relied heavily on outside readings, to a more convenient and educationally useful self-contained text. The Academy regularly updates and revises the course, with the goals of integrating the basic science and clinical practice of ophthalmology and of keeping ophthalmologists current with new developments in the various subspecialties.

The BCSC incorporates the effort and expertise of more than 70 ophthalmologists, organized into 12 section faculties, working with Academy editorial staff. In addition, the course continues to benefit from many lasting contributions made by the faculties of previous editions. Members of the Academy's Practicing Ophthalmologists Advisory Committee for Education serve on each faculty and, as a group, review every volume before and after major revisions.

## Organization of the Course

The 12 sections of the Basic and Clinical Science Course are numbered as follows to reflect a logical order of study, proceeding from fundamental subjects to anatomic subdivisions:

1.  Update on General Medicine
2.  Fundamentals and Principles of Ophthalmology
3.  Optics, Refraction, and Contact Lenses
4.  Ophthalmic Pathology and Intraocular Tumors
5.  Neuro-Ophthalmology
6.  Pediatric Ophthalmology and Strabismus
7.  Orbit, Eyelids, and Lacrimal System
8.  External Disease and Cornea
9.  Intraocular Inflammation and Uveitis
10. Glaucoma
11. Lens and Cataract
12. Retina and Vitreous

In addition, a comprehensive Master Index allows the reader to easily locate subjects throughout the entire series.

## References

Readers who wish to explore specific topics in greater detail may consult the journal references cited within each chapter and the Basic Texts listed at the back of the book. These references are intended to be selective rather than exhaustive, chosen by the BCSC faculty as being important, current, and readily available to residents and practitioners.

Related Academy educational materials are also listed in the appropriate sections. They include books, audiovisual materials, self-assessment programs, clinical modules, and interactive programs.

## Study Questions and CME Credit

Each volume of the BCSC is designed as an independent study activity for ophthalmology residents and practitioners. The learning objectives for this volume are stated on the facing page. The text, illustrations, and references provide the information necessary to achieve the objectives; while the study questions allow readers to test their understanding of the material and their mastery of the objectives. Further, physicians who wish to claim CME credit for this educational activity must complete the study questions and submit the answers, together with the signed Credit Reporting Form and Section Evaluation (these forms are located at the end of the book). Requests for CME credit must be submitted within 3 years of the date of purchase.

## Conclusion

The Basic and Clinical Science Course has expanded greatly over the years, with the addition of much new text and numerous illustrations. Recent editions have sought to place a greater emphasis on clinical applicability, while maintaining a solid foundation in basic science. As with any educational program, it reflects the experience of its authors. As its faculties change and as medicine progresses, new viewpoints are always emerging on controversial subjects and techniques. Not all alternate approaches can be included in this series; as with any educational endeavor, the learner should seek additional sources, including such carefully balanced opinions as the Academy's Preferred Practice Patterns.

The BCSC faculty and staff are continuously striving to improve the educational usefulness of the course; you, the reader, can contribute to this ongoing process. If you have any suggestions or questions about the series, please do not hesitate to contact the faculty or the managing editor.

The authors, editors, and reviewers hope that your study of the BCSC will be of lasting value and that each section will serve as a practical resource for quality patient care.

# OBJECTIVES FOR BCSC SECTION 10

Upon completion of BCSC Section 10, *Glaucoma,* the reader should be able to:

- Identify the epidemiologic features of glaucoma, including the social and economic impacts of the disease
- Summarize recent advances in the understanding of hereditary and genetic factors in glaucoma
- Outline the physiology of aqueous humor dynamics and the control of intraocular pressure (IOP)
- Review the clinical evaluation of the glaucoma patient, including history and general examination, gonioscopy, optic nerve examination, and visual field
- Describe the clinical features of the patient considered a "glaucoma suspect"
- Summarize the clinical features, evaluation, and therapy of primary open-angle glaucoma and normal-tension glaucoma
- List the various clinical features of and therapeutic approaches for the primary and secondary open-angle glaucomas
- Explain the underlying causes of the increased IOP in various forms of secondary open-angle glaucoma and the impact these underlying causes have on management
- Review the mechanisms and pathophysiology of primary angle-closure glaucoma
- Review the pathophysiology of secondary angle-closure glaucoma, both with and without pupillary block
- Outline the pathophysiology and therapy of infantile and juvenile-onset glaucoma
- Differentiate among the various classes of medical therapy for glaucoma, including efficacy, mechanism of action, and safety
- Compare the indications and techniques of various laser and incisional surgical procedures for glaucoma
- Describe cyclodestructive treatment for refractory glaucoma

# Development of Our Concept of Glaucoma and Its Treatment

The word *glaucoma* derives from the Greek word *glaukós,* meaning a watery or diluted blue. Hippocrates mentioned the condition of glaukosis among the infirmities suffered by old people. Hippocrates meant by the term a bluish discoloration of the pupil. The condition was later called *ypochýma* and corresponded to a cataract.

In antiquity glaukosis and hypochyma were considered identical. Later, during the Alexandrian time, glaucoma was thought to be a disease of the crystalline body (or fluid), which changed its normal color to light blue; hypochyma, in contrast, was regarded as the exudation of a fluid that later congealed and lay between the iris and the lens. All glaucomas were considered incurable, while it was believed that some hypochymata could be improved.

The authors of antiquity and Arab physicians interpreted glaucoma as an incurable cataract with desiccation of the lens. During the Middle Ages, the School of Salerno introduced the concept of "gutta serena," which was supposed to be one type of incurable cataract in which the pupil was dilated and clear; the condition was considered to be possibly congenital. According to this school, another type of incurable cataract existed in which the pupil would dilate suddenly and appear green.

Pierre Brisseau, with his little book on cataract and glaucoma published in 1709, was the first to consider glaucoma as a vitreous opacification. He correctly interpreted cataract as an opaque crystalline lens. The first reasonably satisfactory description of glaucoma was written by Charles St. Yves (1722): "Glaucoma is one of the spurious cataracts. First the patients see smoke and fog; then they lose vision while the pupil becomes dilated; finally, only a remnant of vision remains temporally. The disease may begin with severe pain. The prognosis is poor. There is danger that the other eye will also be affected." Quite likely he was describing angle-closure glaucoma.

Johann Zacharias Platner (1745) was the first to state that the glaucomatous eye was hard, resisting the pressure exerted by the fingers. The pressure theory was then emphasized and clarified by William Mackenzie (1830). Jakob Wenzel (1808) thought that glaucoma was primarily a disease of the retina, while S. Canstatt (1831), Julius Sichel (1841), and followers declared glaucoma a form of choroiditis. All of them considered glaucoma incurable. Georg Josef Beer (1817) thought that glaucoma was an opacification of the vitreous and the sequel of an arthritic ophthalmia that would only develop in patients with gout who had had no preceding ocular inflammation.

A few futile attempts were made to treat glaucoma in the early nineteenth century. Mackenzie suggested a sclerotomy or lensectomy. Georg Stromeyer recommended tenotomy of the superior oblique and myotomy of the inferior oblique.

St. Yves wanted to enucleate the affected eye to prevent involvement of the second eye. The first real breakthrough in treatment was the discovery in 1856 by Albrecht von Graefe that iridectomy could be a curative procedure for certain types of glaucoma. He had first tried without success the instillation of atropine and repeated paracenteses to lower intraocular pressure (IOP).

Only with the invention of the ophthalmoscope by Hermann von Helmholtz in 1851 was it possible to observe the changes in the optic nerve head associated with glaucoma. The term *pressure excavation* had been coined by von Graefe. This ophthalmoscopic concept was corroborated by careful pathologic examinations initiated by Heinrich Müller. Edward Jaeger and Isidor Schnabel defended the hypothesis that glaucoma was characterized by specific optic nerve disease.

It soon became obvious that an iridectomy could not cure all types of glaucoma. Albrecht von Graefe had already noted that a "cystoid scar," meaning a filtering bleb in today's jargon, would offer certain advantages for normalizing IOP. Sclerotomy was first proposed by Louis de Wecker in 1869. Surgeons then tried to keep the wound open on purpose, either by infolding of the conjunctiva (H. Herbert, 1903) or by incarceration of the iris (George Critchett of London in 1858 and Soren Holth of Oslo in 1904). Finally, the iridosclerectomy was devised by Pierre Lagrange in Paris (1905), and the trephining operation was introduced by Robert H. Elliot of Madras, India. Thermosclerotomy was first described by Luigi Preziosi of Malta in 1924, and it was later modified and popularized by Harold Scheie of Philadelphia in 1958. Trabeculectomy was subsequently described by Watson and Cairns in the 1950s in England.

The medical treatment of glaucoma was initiated with eserine, which is derived from the Calabar bean of West Africa. This drug was first recognized as a miotic and used for treating iris prolapse. In 1876 Ludwig Laqueur of Strasbourg and Adolf Weber of Darmstadt were the first to use eserine to treat glaucoma. The alkaloid pilocarpine was isolated in 1875, and it was first topically applied to the eye by John Tweedy of London (1875) and by Weber (1876) in an effort to lower IOP.

Frederick C. Blodi, MD

# CHAPTER I

# Introduction to Glaucoma: Terminology, Epidemiology, and Heredity

## Definitions

The term *glaucoma* refers to a group of diseases that have in common a characteristic *optic neuropathy* with associated *visual field loss* for which elevated *intraocular pressure (IOP)* is one of the primary risk factors. The commonly accepted range for normal IOP in the general population is 10–22 mm Hg. Three factors determine the IOP (Fig I-1):

☐ The rate of aqueous humor production by the ciliary body

☐ Resistance to aqueous outflow across the trabecular meshwork–Schlemm's canal system

☐ The level of episcleral venous pressure

In most cases increased IOP is caused by increased resistance to aqueous humor outflow.

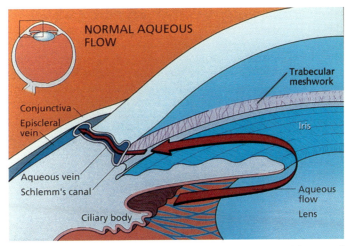

FIG I-1—Diagrammatic cross section of the anterior segment of the normal eye, showing the site of aqueous production (ciliary body) and sites of resistance to aqueous outflow (trabecular meshwork–Schlemm's canal system and episcleral venous plexus).

Several risk factors, many of which remain unknown, increase the likelihood of the development of glaucoma. Those factors known to be associated with an increased risk for the development of glaucoma besides increased IOP include advanced age, racial background, and a positive family history.

In most individuals the optic nerve and visual field changes seen in glaucoma are determined by both the level of the IOP and the resistance of the optic nerve axons to pressure damage. Other factors, which at present are poorly defined, also seem to predispose the optic nerve axons to damage. Although progressive changes in the visual field and optic nerve are usually related to increased IOP, in cases of normal-tension glaucoma the IOP remains within the normal range (see chapter IV). In most cases of glaucoma the IOP is too high for proper functioning of the optic nerve axons, and lowering the IOP will stabilize the damage. In cases involving other pathophysiologic mechanisms that may affect the optic nerve, however, progression of optic nerve damage may continue despite lowering of IOP.

The terms *primary* and *secondary* have been helpful in current definitions of glaucoma, and they are still in widespread use. However, as discussed below under Classification, new concepts are emerging that may change this common usage. By definition, the *primary glaucomas* are not associated with known ocular or systemic disorders that cause increased resistance to aqueous outflow. The primary glaucomas usually affect both eyes and may be inherited. Conversely, the *secondary glaucomas* are associated with ocular or systemic disorders responsible for decreased aqueous outflow. The diseases that cause secondary glaucoma are often unilateral, and familial occurrence is less common.

## Classification

### Open-Angle, Angle-Closure, Primary, and Secondary Glaucomas

Traditionally, glaucoma has been classified as open angle or closed angle and as primary or secondary (Table I-1). Differentiation of open-angle glaucoma from closed-angle glaucoma is essential from a therapeutic standpoint (see chapters IV and V). The concept of primary and secondary glaucomas is also useful, but it reflects our lack of understanding of the pathophysiologic mechanisms underlying the glaucomatous process. Open-angle glaucoma is classified as primary when no identifiable underlying cause of the events that led to outflow obstruction and elevation of IOP can be found. It is classified as secondary when an abnormality is identified and a putative role in the pathogenesis can be ascribed to this abnormality.

However, it is now recognized that all glaucomas are secondary to some abnormality, whether currently identified or not. As our knowledge of the mechanisms underlying the causes of glaucoma continues to expand, the primary/secondary classification has become increasingly artificial. This scheme is particularly inadequate for classifying the angle-closure glaucomas.

Other schemes for classifying glaucoma have been proposed. Classification of the glaucomas based on initial events and on mechanisms of outflow obstruction are two schemes that have gained increasing popularity (Table I-2).

Ritch R, Shields MB, Krupin T, eds. *The Glaucomas.* 2nd ed. St Louis: Mosby; 1996:722.

TABLE I-1

CLASSIFICATION OF GLAUCOMA

| TYPE | CHARACTERISTICS |
|------|-----------------|
| **Open-angle glaucoma** (Fig I-2, see p 9) | |
| Primary open-angle glaucoma (POAG) | Not associated with known ocular or systemic disorders that cause increased resistance to aqueous outflow or damage to optic nerve; usually associated with elevated IOP |
| Normal-tension glaucoma | Considered in continuum of POAG; terminology often used when IOP is not elevated |
| Juvenile open-angle glaucoma | Terminology often used when open-angle glaucoma diagnosed at young age (typically 10–30 years of age) |
| Glaucoma suspect | Normal optic disc and visual field associated with elevated IOP |
| | Suspicious optic disc and/or visual field with normal IOP |
| Secondary open-angle glaucoma | Increased resistance to trabecular meshwork outflow associated with other conditions (e.g., pigmentary glaucoma, phacolytic glaucoma, steroid-induced glaucoma) |
| | Increased posttrabecular resistance to outflow secondary to elevated episcleral venous pressure (e.g., carotid cavernous sinus fistula) |
| **Angle-closure glaucoma** (Fig I-3, see p 9) | |
| Primary angle-closure glaucoma with relative pupillary block | Movement of aqueous humor from posterior chamber to anterior chamber restricted; peripheral iris in contact with trabecular meshwork |
| Acute angle closure | Occurs when IOP rises rapidly as a result of relatively sudden blockage of the trabecular meshwork |
| Subacute angle closure (intermittent angle closure) | Repeated, brief episodes of angle closure with mild symptoms and elevated IOP, often a prelude to acute angle closure |
| Chronic angle closure | IOP elevation caused by variable portions of anterior chamber angle being permanently closed by peripheral anterior synechiae |
| Secondary angle-closure glaucoma with pupillary block | (E.g., swollen lens, secluded pupil) |
| Secondary angle-closure glaucoma without pupillary block | Posterior pushing mechanism: lens–iris diaphragm pushed forward (e.g., posterior segment tumor, scleral buckling procedure, uveal effusion) |
| | Anterior pulling mechanism: anterior segment process pulling iris forward to form peripheral anterior synechiae (e.g., iridocorneal endothelial syndrome, neovascular glaucoma, inflammation) |
| Plateau iris syndrome | Primary angle closure with or without component of pupillary block, but pupillary block is not predominant mechanism of angle closure |
| **Childhood glaucoma** | |
| Primary congenital/ infantile glaucoma | Primary glaucoma present from birth to first few years of life |
| Glaucoma associated with congenital anomalies | Associated with ocular disorders (e.g., anterior segment dysgenesis, aniridia) |
| | Associated with systemic disorders (e.g., rubella, Lowe syndrome) |
| Secondary glaucoma in infants and children | (E.g., glaucoma secondary to retinoblastoma or trauma) |

TABLE 1-2

Classification of the Glaucomas Based on Mechanisms of Outflow Obstruction*

| OPEN-ANGLE GLAUCOMA MECHANISMS | | | ANGLE-CLOSURE GLAUCOMA MECHANISMS | | DEVELOPMENTAL ANOMALIES OF ANTERIOR CHAMBER ANGLE |
|---|---|---|---|---|---|
| PRETRABECULAR (MEMBRANE OVERGROWTH) | TRABECULAR | POSTTRABECULAR | ANTERIOR ("PULLING") | POSTERIOR ("PUSHING") | |
| Fibrovascular membrane (neovascular glaucoma) | Idiopathic | Obstruction of Schlemm's canal, e.g., collapse at canal | Contracture of membranes | With pupillary block | Incomplete development of trabecular meshwork/ Schlemm's canal |
| Endothelial layer, often with Descemet-like membrane | Chronic open-angle glaucoma | Elevated episcleral venous pressure | Neovascular glaucoma | Pupillary-block glaucoma | Congenital (infantile) glaucoma |
| Iridocorneal endothelial syndrome | Juvenile open-angle glaucoma | Carotid cavernous fistula | Iridocorneal endothelial syndrome | Lens-induced mechanisms | Axenfeld-Rieger syndrome |
| Posterior polymorphous dystrophy | "Clogging" of trabecular meshwork | Cavernous sinus thrombosis | Posterior polymorphous dystrophy | Phacomorphic lens | Peters anomaly |
| Penetrating and non-penetrating trauma | Red blood cells | Retrobulbar tumors | Penetrating and non-penetrating trauma | Ectopia lentis | Glaucomas associated with other developmental anomalies |
| Epithelial downgrowth | Hemorrhagic glaucoma | Thyroid ophthalmopathy | Consolidation of inflammatory products | Posterior synechiae | Iridocorneal adhesions |
| Fibrous ingrowth | Ghost cell glaucoma | Superior vena cava obstruction | | Iris–vitreous block | Broad strands (Axenfeld-Rieger syndrome) |
| Inflammatory membrane | Sickled red blood cells | Mediastinal tumors | | Pseudophakia | Fine strands that contract to close angle (aniridia) |
| Fuchs heterochromic iridocyclitis | Macrophages | Sturge-Weber syndrome | | Uveitis | |
| Luetic interstitial keratitis | Hemolytic glaucoma | Familial episcleral venous pressure elevation | | Without pupillary block | |
| | Phacolytic glaucoma | | | Ciliary block (malignant) glaucoma | |
| | Melanomalytic glaucoma | | | Lens-induced mechanisms | |
| | Neoplastic cells | | | Phacomorphic lens | |
| | Primary ocular tumors | | | Ectopia lentis | |
| | Neoplastic tumors | | | Following lens extraction (forward vitreous shift) | |
| | Juvenile xanthogranuloma | | | Anterior rotation of ciliary body | |
| | Pigment particles | | | Following scleral buckling | |
| | Pigmentary glaucoma | | | Following panretinal photocoagulation | |
| | Exfoliation syndrome (glaucoma capsulare) | | | Central retinal vein occlusion | |
| | Malignant melanoma | | | Intraocular tumors | |
| | Protein | | | Malignant melanoma | |
| | Uveitis | | | Retinoblastoma | |
| | Lens-induced glaucoma | | | Cysts of the iris and ciliary body | |
| | Viscoelastic agents | | | Retrolenticular tissue contracture | |
| | α-chymotrypsin–induced glaucoma | | | Retinopathy of prematurity (retrolental fibroplasia) | |
| | Vitreous | | | Persistent hyperplastic primary vitreous | |
| | Alterations of the trabecular meshwork | | | | |
| | Steroid-induced glaucoma | | | | |
| | Edema | | | | |
| | Uveitis (trabeculitis) | | | | |
| | Scleritis and episcleritis | | | | |
| | Alkali burns | | | | |
| | Trauma (angle recession) | | | | |
| | Intraocular foreign bodies (hemosiderosis, chalcosis) | | | | |

PLATEAU IRIS SYNDROME

*Clinical examples cited in this table do not represent an inclusive list of the glaucomas.
Modified with permission from Ritch R, Shields MB, Krupin T, eds. *The Glaucomas.* 2nd ed. St Louis; Mosby; 1996:722.

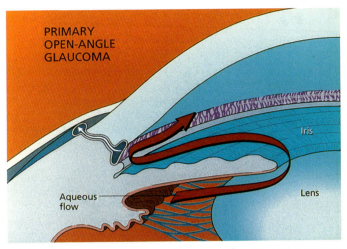

FIG I-2—Schematic of open-angle glaucoma with resistance to aqueous outflow through the trabecular meshwork–Schlemm's canal system in the absence of gross anatomic obstruction. Small white arrow shows normal path of outflow and indicates that resistance in this illustration is relative, not total.

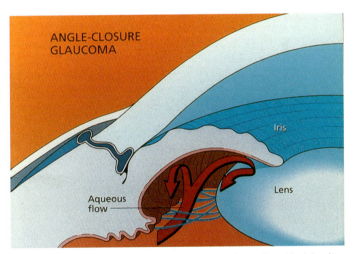

FIG I-3—Schematic of angle-closure glaucoma with pupillary block leading to peripheral iris obstruction of the trabecular meshwork.

*Combined-Mechanism Glaucoma*

When a combination of two or more forms of glaucoma present either sequentially or simultaneously, the term *combined-mechanism glaucoma* is sometimes used. This situation may occur following a primary acute angle-closure glaucoma attack, when IOP remains elevated after a peripheral iridectomy in spite of an open and normal-appearing anterior chamber angle. Combined-mechanism glaucoma can also appear in a patient with open-angle glaucoma who develops secondary angle closure from other causes. Examples include a patient with open-angle glaucoma who develops angle closure as a result of miotic therapy or a patient with pseudophakic open-angle glaucoma who develops peripheral anterior synechiae after an episode of pupillary block.

IOP elevation in these cases can occur as a result of either or both of the following:

□ The intrinsic resistance of the trabecular meshwork to aqueous outflow in open-angle glaucoma

□ The direct anatomic obstruction of the filtering meshwork by synechiae in angle-closure glaucoma

Treatment is modified based on the proportion of open angle to closed angle and the etiology of the angle-closure component.

## Epidemiologic Aspects of Glaucoma

*Primary Open-Angle Glaucoma*

**Magnitude of the problem**   Primary open-angle glaucoma represents a significant public health problem. At least 2.25 million individuals in the United States 45 years of age or older are estimated to have this disease. Estimates based on the available data indicate that between 84,000 and 116,000 of them have become bilaterally blind (best-corrected visual acuity less than or equal to 20/200 or visual field <20°). POAG is thus an important cause of blindness in the United States and the most frequent cause of nonreversible blindness in black Americans.

The World Health Organization (WHO) has undertaken an extensive analysis of the literature to estimate the prevalence, incidence, and severity of the different types of glaucoma on a worldwide basis. Using data collected predominantly in the late 1980s and early 1990s, WHO estimated the global population of people with high IOP (>21 mm Hg) at 104.5 million. The incidence of primary open-angle glaucoma was estimated at 2.4 million people per year. Blindness prevalence for all types of glaucoma was estimated at 5.2 million people, with 3 million cases caused by POAG. The different types of glaucoma were theoretically calculated to be responsible for 15% of blindness, placing glaucoma as the third leading cause of blindness worldwide, following cataract and trachoma.

Despite these staggering statistics, the impact of glaucoma from a public health perspective has not been fully appreciated. Relatively little information is currently available regarding the individual burden associated with the psychologic effects of having a potentially blinding chronic disease, the debilitating side effects of treatment, and the qualitative functional loss associated with diminished visual fields. Nor does reliable information exist on the societal costs associated with the detection, treatment, and rehabilitation of this disease.

***Prevalence***   Prevalence of POAG shows a strong racial disparity. Among whites 40 years of age and older, a prevalence of between 1.1% and 2.1% has been consistently obtained by population-based studies performed throughout the world. The prevalence among blacks is three to four times higher. The prevalence of POAG increases with age, and estimates among persons in their seventies have generally been three to eight times higher compared with persons in their forties.

***Risk factors***   Identifying risk factors is important because this information may lead to development of strategies for disease screening and prevention and may be useful in identifying persons for whom close medical supervision is indicated. Strictly defined, a factor can be considered a risk factor only if it predates disease occurrence. From a clinical perspective, it is often difficult to differentiate very early disease from normal. In fact, this determination is often dependent on how the disease is defined.

Glaucoma is usually defined by the presence of characteristic visual field defects and sometimes, in the absence of visual field defects, by the appearance of optic nerve damage. How often this diagnosis is made in marginal cases is influenced by the sensitivity of available diagnostic tests. Thus, it may be difficult to determine whether abnormalities in certain parameters—e.g., optic nerve parameters such as nerve fiber layer loss—are indicative of increased susceptibility to developing glaucoma or are signs of early disease. From a practical standpoint, the distinction is unimportant. Individuals manifesting such abnormalities must be closely monitored for signs of clinically significant disease development in either situation.

The quality of available data regarding potential risk factors for the development of POAG varies greatly. Evidence that IOP, age, race, and positive family history are risk factors for POAG is considerable and reliable. Data also support diabetes and myopia as risk factors, but these data are generally less convincing. The relevance of sex and of various systemic factors, such as systemic hypertension and arteriosclerotic and ischemic vascular disease, to glaucoma risk has been widely debated, and currently available data do not permit the drawing of definitive conclusions.

## Primary Angle-Closure Glaucoma

Compared with primary open-angle glaucoma, the epidemiology of primary angle-closure glaucoma (PACG) has received much less attention. Most of the available information is derived from hospital-based surveys or from population screenings of small high-risk subpopulations.

***Race***   The prevalence of primary angle-closure glaucoma varies in different racial and ethnic groups. Among white populations in the United States and Europe, it is estimated at approximately 0.1%. Inuit populations from Arctic regions have the highest known prevalence of primary angle-closure glaucoma, 20–40 times higher than whites. The relative prevalences of PACG and POAG among Inuits are also the reverse of what is noted in white populations, with POAG being uncommon.

Estimates of the prevalence of primary angle-closure glaucoma in Asian populations have varied considerably. Some of this variability may be the result of differences in quality and design of the studies from which the estimates were derived. Another factor, however, is that Asian populations are not one homogeneous group, and substantial differences in PACG prevalence between many Asian groups are likely. The available data suggest that most of the Asian population groups have a prevalence of primary angle-closure glaucoma between that of whites and Inuits.

Acute angle-closure glaucoma is relatively uncommon in blacks. However, chronic angle-closure glaucoma is much more common than initially believed. Some studies have suggested that the prevalence of primary angle-closure glaucoma in blacks is similar to that in whites, with most of the cases in blacks being of the chronic variety.

***Sex*** Women of all races develop acute angle-closure glaucoma three to four times more often than do men. Studies of normal eyes have shown that women have shallower anterior chambers than men.

***Age*** The anterior chamber decreases in depth and volume with age. These changes predispose to pupillary block, and the prevalence of pupillary-block angle-closure glaucoma thus increases with age. Acute angle-closure glaucoma is most common between the ages of 55 and 65 years, but it can occur in young adults and the elderly and has been reported in children.

***Refraction*** The anterior chamber depth and volume are smaller in hyperopic eyes. Although primary angle-closure glaucoma may occur in eyes with any type of refractive error, it is thus typically associated with hyperopia.

***Inheritance*** Some of the anatomic features of the eye that predispose to pupillary block, such as more forward position of the lens and greater than average lens thickness, are inherited. Thus relatives of subjects with angle-closure glaucoma are at greater risk of developing angle-closure than the general population. However, estimates of the exact risk vary greatly.

Epstein DL, Allingham RR, Schuman JS, eds. *Chandler and Grant's Glaucoma.* 4th ed. Baltimore: Williams & Wilkins; 1997:641–646.

Ritch R, Shields MB, Krupin T, eds. *The Glaucomas.* 2nd ed. St Louis: Mosby; 1996: 753–765.

## Hereditary and Genetic Factors

The prevalences of glaucoma, enlarged cup–disc ratio, and elevated IOP are all much higher in siblings and offspring of patients with glaucoma than in the general population. A positive family history is a major risk factor for the development of POAG. The prevalence of glaucoma among siblings of patients is approximately 10%, and the lifetime absolute risk of glaucoma at age 89 years is 10 times higher for relatives of glaucoma patients compared with relatives of unaffected persons.

The precise mechanism of inheritance is not clear, and a single underlying susceptibility gene cannot be assumed. Inheritance may involve more that one gene (polygenic), have a late or variable age of onset, demonstrate incomplete penetrance (the disease may not develop even when the causative gene has been inherited), and may have substantial environmental influences. See also BCSC Section 2, *Fundamentals and Principles of Ophthalmology,* Part 3, Genetics.

Genetic studies have been successful in identifying the location of genes for juvenile open-angle glaucoma (chromosome 1q21–q31) and for disorders associat-

## TABLE I-3

### CLONED GENES KNOWN TO BE ASSOCIATED WITH GLAUCOMA

| GENE | LOCUS | PHENOTYPE |
|---|---|---|
| TIGR/Myocilin | 1q23 (GLC1A) | Juvenile and adult open-angle glaucoma |
| CYP1B1 | 2p21 (GLC3A) | Congenital glaucoma |
| PITX2 | 4q25 (RIEG1) | Rieger syndrome |
| FKHL7 | 6p25 (IDYS1) | Iridodysgenesis |
| LMX1B | 9q34 (NPS1) | Glaucoma associated with nail-patella syndrome |
| PAX6 | 11p13 (AN1) | Aniridia |

Table courtesy of Janey L. Wiggs, MD, PhD.

ed with glaucoma such as Axenfeld-Rieger syndrome (4q25 or 4q27) (Table I-3). Identifying the gene(s) responsible for POAG will revolutionize our understanding of this disorder and will lead to major new therapeutic interventions.

Wolfs RC, Klaver CC, Ramrattan RS, et al. Genetic risk of primary open-angle glaucoma: population-based familial aggregation study. *Arch Ophthalmol.* 1998;116: 1640–1645.

# CHAPTER II

# Intraocular Pressure and Aqueous Humor Dynamics

The clinical approach to glaucoma begins with an understanding of *aqueous humor,* which flows from the posterior chamber through the pupil into the anterior chamber and exits the eye by passing through the *trabecular meshwork* into *Schlemm's canal* and then draining into the venous system through a plexus of collector channels, as shown in Figure I-1. The formation and outflow of aqueous humor are discussed in detail below. The *Goldmann equation* summarizes the relationship between these factors and the IOP in the undisturbed eye:

$$P_0 = (F/C) + P_v$$

in which $P_0$ is the IOP in millimeters of mercury (mm Hg), F is the rate of aqueous formation in microliters per minute ($\mu$l/min), C is the facility of outflow in microliters per minute per millimeter of mercury ($\mu$l/min/mm Hg), and $P_v$ is the episcleral venous pressure in millimeters of mercury. Resistance to outflow (R) is the inverse of facility (C) and may replace C in rearrangements of the Goldmann equation.

## Aqueous Humor Formation

Aqueous humor is formed by the *ciliary processes,* each of which is composed of a double layer of epithelium over a core of stroma and a rich supply of fenestrated capillaries (Fig II-1). The apical surfaces of both the outer pigmented and the inner nonpigmented layers of epithelium face each other and are joined by tight junctions, which are probably an important part of the blood–aqueous barrier. The inner non-pigmented epithelial cells contain numerous mitochondria and microvilli, and these cells are thought to be the site of aqueous production. The ciliary processes provide a large surface area for secretion. BCSC Section 2, *Fundamentals and Principles of Ophthalmology,* discusses aqueous humor composition in detail in Part 4, Biochemistry and Metabolism.

Aqueous humor formation is not precisely understood, but it involves the combination of several processes:

□ Active transport (secretion)

□ Ultrafiltration

□ Simple diffusion

*Active transport* consumes energy to move substances against an electrochemical gradient and is independent of pressure. The identity of the precise ion or ions transported is not known, but sodium, chloride, and bicarbonate are involved. Active transport accounts for the majority of aqueous production and involves, at least in part, activity of the enzyme carbonic anhydrase II. *Ultrafiltration* refers to a pressure-

Posterior Chamber

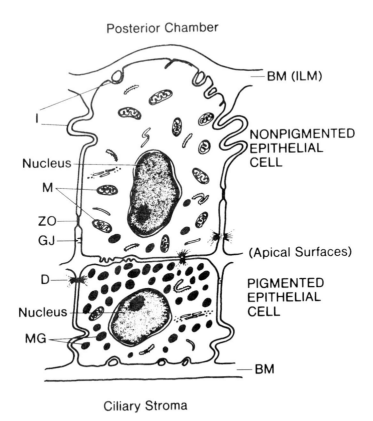

FIG II-1—The two layers of the ciliary epithelium showing apical surfaces in apposition to each other. Basement membrane *(BM)* lines the double layer and constitutes the internal limiting membrane *(ILM)* on the inner surface. The nonpigmented epithelium is characterized by mitochondria *(M)*, zonulae occludens *(ZO)*, and lateral and surface interdigitations *(I)*. The pigmented epithelium contains numerous melanin granules *(MG)*. Additional intercellular junctions include desmosomes *(D)* and gap junctions *(GJ)*. (Reproduced with permission from Shields MB. *Textbook of Glaucoma.* 3rd ed. Baltimore: Williams & Wilkins; 1992.)

dependent movement along a pressure gradient. In the ciliary processes the hydrostatic pressure difference between capillary pressure and IOP favors fluid movement into the eye, while the oncotic gradient between the two resists fluid movement. The relationship between secretion and ultrafiltration is not known. *Diffusion* is the passive movement of ions across a membrane related to charge.

## Suppression of Aqueous Formation

The mechanisms of action of the classes of drugs that suppress aqueous formation—the *carbonic anhydrase inhibitors, beta-adrenergic antagonists (beta blockers),* and *alpha$_2$ agonists*—are also not precisely understood. The role of the enzyme carbonic anhydrase has been debated vigorously. Evidence suggests that the bicarbonate ion is actively secreted in human eyes; thus, the function of the enzyme may be to provide this ion. Carbonic anhydrase may also provide bicarbonate or hydrogen ions for an intracellular buffering system.

Current evidence indicates that beta$_2$ receptors are the most prevalent adrenergic receptors in the ciliary epithelium. The significance of this finding is unclear, but beta-adrenergic antagonists may affect active transport by causing a decrease in either the efficiency of the Na$^+$/K$^+$ pump or in the number of pump sites. For a detailed discussion and illustration of the sodium pump and pump/leak mechanism, see BCSC Section 2, *Fundamentals and Principles of Ophthalmology*, and BCSC Section 11, *Lens and Cataract*.

### Rate of Aqueous Formation

The most common method used to measure the rate of aqueous formation is *fluorophotometry*. Fluorescein is administered systemically or topically, and the subsequent decline in its anterior chamber concentration is measured optically and used to calculate aqueous flow. Normal flow is approximately 2–3 μl/min, or a 1% turnover in aqueous volume per minute.

Aqueous formation varies diurnally and drops during sleep. It also decreases with age, as does outflow facility. The rate of aqueous formation is affected by a variety of factors:

□ The integrity of the blood–aqueous barrier

□ Blood flow to the ciliary body

□ Neurohumoral regulation of vascular tissue and the ciliary epithelium

Aqueous inflow falls when the eye is injured or inflamed and following the administration of certain drugs such as general anesthetics and some systemic hypotensive agents. Carotid occlusive disease may also decrease aqueous humor production.

## Aqueous Humor Outflow

The facility of outflow (C in the Goldmann equation; see page 14) varies widely in normal eyes. The mean value reported ranges from 0.22 to 0.28 μl/min/mm Hg. Outflow facility decreases with age and is affected by surgery, trauma, medications, and endocrine factors. Patients with glaucoma and elevated IOP have decreased outflow facility.

### Trabecular Outflow

Most of the aqueous humor exits the eye by way of the trabecular meshwork–Schlemm's canal–venous system. The trabecular meshwork can be divided into three zones (Fig II-2):

□ Uveal

□ Corneoscleral

□ Juxtacanalicular

The primary resistance to outflow occurs at the juxtacanalicular tissue.

The trabecular meshwork functions as a one-way valve that permits aqueous to leave the eye by bulk flow but limits flow in the other direction independently of

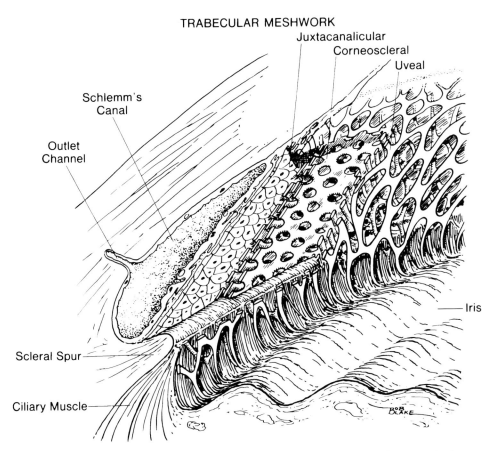

TRABECULAR MESHWORK

FIG II-2—Three layers of trabecular meshwork (shown in cutaway views): uveal, corneoscleral, and juxtacanalicular. (Reproduced with permission from Shields MB. *Textbook of Glaucoma.* 3rd ed. Baltimore: Williams & Wilkins; 1992.)

energy. Aqueous moves both across and between the endothelial cells lining the inner wall of Schlemm's canal. Once in Schlemm's canal, aqueous enters the episcleral venous plexus by way of scleral collector channels. When IOP is low, the trabecular meshwork may collapse, or proteins and blood cells may reflux into Schlemm's canal and be visible on gonioscopy.

### Uveoscleral Outflow

In the normal eye any nontrabecular outflow is termed *uveoscleral outflow.* A variety of mechanisms are involved, predominantly aqueous passage from the anterior chamber into the ciliary muscle and then into the supraciliary and suprachoroidal spaces. The fluid then exits the eye through the intact sclera or along the nerves and the vessels that penetrate it. Uveoscleral outflow is pressure-independent and is believed to be influenced by age. Recent research suggests that it may be a more important route of aqueous outflow than previously thought, possibly accounting for up to 50% in normal eyes of young people. It is increased by cycloplegic, adrenergic, and prostaglandin agents and certain forms of surgery (e.g., cyclodialysis) and is decreased by miotics.

## Tonography

The ease with which aqueous can leave the eye is measured by tonography as the facility of outflow. This measurement can be taken using a Schiøtz tonometer of known weight, which is placed on the cornea, suddenly elevating IOP. The rate at which the pressure declines with time is related to the ease with which the aqueous leaves the eye. The decline in IOP over time can be used to determine outflow facility in $\mu$l/min/mm Hg through a series of mathematical calculations.

Unfortunately, tonography depends on a number of assumptions (e.g., the elastic properties of the eye, stability of aqueous formation, constancy of ocular blood volume) and is subject to many sources of error (e.g., calibration problems, patient fixation, eyelid squeezing, technician errors). These problems reduce the accuracy and reproducibility of tonography for an individual patient. At present, tonography is best used as a research tool for the investigation of matters such as drug effects. It is rarely used clinically.

## Episcleral Venous Pressure

Episcleral venous pressure is relatively stable, except when alterations in body position and certain diseases of the orbit, head, and neck obstruct venous return to the heart or shunt blood from the arterial to the venous system. The usual range of values is 8–12 mm Hg. The pressure in the episcleral veins can be measured with specialized equipment. In acute conditions IOP rises approximately 1 mm Hg for every 1 mm Hg increase in episcleral venous pressure. The relationship is more complex, however, in chronic conditions. Chronic elevations of episcleral venous pressure may be accompanied by changes in IOP that are of greater, lesser, or the same magnitude.

## Intraocular Pressure

### Distribution in the Population and Relation to Glaucoma

Pooled data from large epidemiologic studies indicate that the mean IOP is approximately 16 mm Hg, with a standard deviation of 3 mm Hg. IOP, however, has a non-gaussian distribution with a skew toward higher pressures, especially in individuals over age 40 (Fig II-3). The value 21 mm Hg has been used in the past both to separate normal and abnormal pressures and to define which patients required ocular hypotensive therapy. This division was based largely on the erroneous assumptions that glaucomatous damage is caused exclusively by pressures that are higher than normal and that normal pressures do not cause damage.

General agreement has now been reached that, for the population as a whole, no clear line exists between safe and unsafe IOP: some eyes undergo damage at IOPs of 18 mm Hg or less, while others tolerate IOPs in the 30s. However, IOP is still seen as a very important risk factor for the development of glaucomatous damage. Although other risk factors affect an individual's susceptibility to glaucomatous damage, IOP is the only one that can be altered at this time.

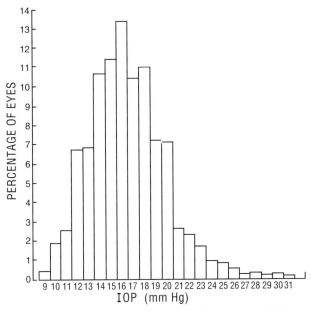

FIG II-3—Frequency distribution of intraocular pressure: 5220 eyes in the Framingham Eye Study. (Reproduced from Colton T, Ederer F. The distribution of intraocular pressures in the general population. *Surv Ophthalmol.* 1980;25:123–129.)

### Factors Influencing Intraocular Pressure

IOP varies with a number of factors, including the following:

□ Time of day

□ Heartbeat

□ Respiration

□ Exercise

□ Fluid intake

□ Systemic medications

□ Topical drugs

Alcohol consumption results in a transient decrease in IOP. Caffeine may cause a small, transient rise in IOP. Cannabis decreases IOP but has not been proved clinically useful. IOP is higher when the patient is recumbent rather than upright. Some people have an exaggerated rise in IOP when they lie down, and this tendency may be important in the pathogenesis of some forms of glaucoma. IOP usually increases with age and is genetically influenced: higher pressures are more common in relatives of patients with primary open-angle glaucoma than in the general population.

## Diurnal Variation

In normal individuals IOP varies 2–6 mm Hg over a 24-hour period, as aqueous humor production changes. The higher the pressure, the greater the fluctuation, and a diurnal fluctuation of greater than 10 mm Hg is suggestive of glaucoma. Many people reach their peak pressures in the morning hours, but others do so in the afternoon or evening, and still others follow no reproducible pattern. To detect such fluctuations, ocular pressure is measured at multiple times around the clock. These measurements can sometimes be useful in evaluating suspected normal-tension glaucoma, assessing the effect that therapy changes have on pressure control, and determining why optic nerve damage might occur despite apparently good control of pressure.

## Clinical Measurement of Intraocular Pressure

Measurement of IOP in a clinical setting requires a force that indents or flattens the eye. *Applanation tonometry* is the method used most widely. It is based on the Imbert-Fick principle, which states that the pressure inside an ideal dry, thin-walled sphere equals the force necessary to flatten its surface divided by the area of the flattening:

$$P = F/A \text{ (where } P = \text{pressure, } F = \text{force, } A = \text{area)}$$

In applanation tonometry the cornea is flattened, and IOP is determined by measuring the applanating force and the area flattened (Fig II-4).

The *Goldmann applanation tonometer* measures the force necessary to flatten an area of the cornea of 3.06 mm diameter. At this diameter the resistance of the cornea to flattening is counterbalanced by the capillary attraction of the tear film meniscus for the tonometer head. Furthermore, the IOP (in mm Hg) equals the flattening force (in grams) multiplied by 10. A split-image prism allows the examiner to determine the flattened area with great accuracy. Fluorescein in the tear film is used to outline the area of flattening. The semicircles move with the ocular pulse, and the end point is reached when the inner edges of the semicircles touch each other at the midpoint of their excursion (Fig II-5).

Applanation measurements are safe, easy to perform, and relatively accurate in most clinical situations. Of the currently available devices, the Goldmann applanation tonometer is the most valid and reliable. Since applanation does not displace much fluid (approximately 0.5 μl) or substantially increase the pressure in the eye, this method is relatively unaffected by ocular rigidity. Possible sources of error, however, include

□ Squeezing of the eyelids

□ Breath holding or Valsalva's maneuvers

□ Pressure on the globe

□ Extraocular muscle force applied to a restricted globe

□ Tight collars

□ An inaccurately calibrated tonometer

Excessive fluorescein results in wide mires and an inaccurately high reading, whereas inadequate fluorescein leads to low readings.

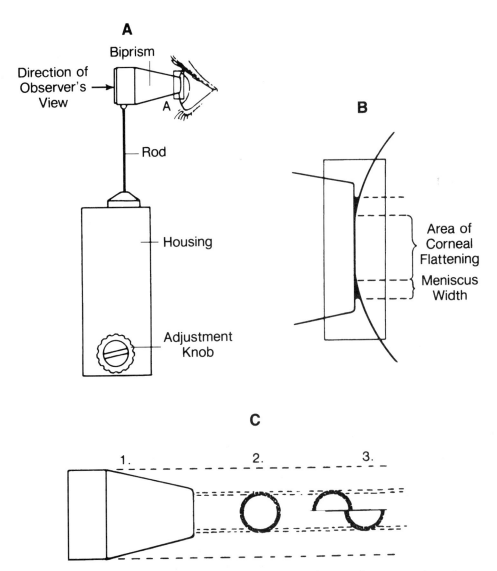

**A**

Biprism

Direction of
Observer's
View →

A

Rod

Housing

Adjustment
Knob

**B**

Area of
Corneal
Flattening

Meniscus
Width

**C**

1.          2.          3.

FIG II-4—Goldmann-type applanation tonometry. *A,* Basic features of tonometer, shown in contact with patient's cornea. *B,* Enlargement shows tear film meniscus created by contact of biprism and cornea. *C,* View through biprism *(1)* reveals circular meniscus *(2),* which is converted into semicircle (3) by prisms. (Reproduced with permission from Shields MB. *Textbook of Glaucoma.* 3rd ed. Baltimore: Williams & Wilkins; 1992.)

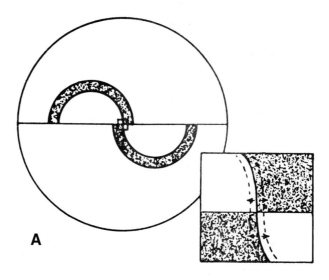

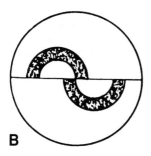

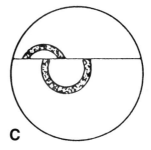

FIG II-5—Semicircles of Goldmann-type applanation tonometer. *A,* Proper width and position. Enlargement depicts excursions of semicircles caused by ocular pulsations. *B,* Semicircles are too wide. *C,* Improper vertical and horizontal alignment. (Reproduced with permission from Shields MB. *Textbook of Glaucoma.* 3rd ed. Baltimore: Williams & Wilkins; 1992.)

Marked corneal astigmatism causes an elliptical fluorescein pattern. To obtain an accurate reading, the clinician should rotate the prism so that the red mark on the prism holder is set at the least curved meridian of the cornea (along the negative axis). Alternately, two pressure readings taken 90° apart can be averaged.

The accuracy of applanation tonometry is reduced in certain situations. Corneal edema predisposes to inaccurately low readings, whereas pressure measurements taken over a corneal scar will be falsely high. Tonometry performed over a soft contact lens gives falsely low values. Alterations in scleral rigidity may compromise the accuracy of measurements; for example, applanation readings that follow scleral buckling procedures may be inaccurately low.

Applanation tonometry measurements are also affected by the central corneal thickness. Increased central corneal thickness may give an artificially high and decreased central corneal thickness may give an artificially low IOP measurement. IOP measured after photorefractive keratectomy (PRK) and laser in situ keratomileusis (LASIK) may be reduced because of changes in the corneal thickness induced by these and other refractive procedures.

The *Perkins tonometer* is a counterbalanced tonometer that is portable and can be used with the patient either upright or supine. It is similar to the Goldmann tonometer in using a split-image device and fluorescein staining of the tears.

**Methods other than Goldmann-type applanation tonometry**   *Noncontact (air-puff) tonometers* measure IOP without touching the eye, by measuring the time necessary for a given force of air to flatten a given area of the cornea. Readings obtained with these instruments vary widely, and they often overestimate IOP. These instruments are often used in large-scale glaucoma-screening programs or by nonmedical health care providers.

The group of *portable electronic applanation* devices (e.g., Tonopen) that applanate a very small area of the cornea are particularly useful in the presence of corneal scars or edema. The *pneumatic tonometer* has a pressure-sensing device that consists of a gas-filled chamber covered by a Silastic diaphragm. The gas in the chamber escapes through an exhaust vent. As the diaphragm touches the cornea, the gas vent is reduced in size and the pressure in the chamber rises. Because this instrument, too, applanates only a small area of the cornea, it is especially useful in the presence of corneal scars or edema.

*Schiøtz tonometry* determines IOP by measuring the indentation of the cornea produced by a known weight. The indentation is read on a linear scale on the instrument and is converted to mm Hg by a calibration table. Because of a number of practical and theoretical problems, however, Schiøtz tonometry is now rarely used.

It is possible to estimate IOP by *digital pressure* on the globe. This test may be used with uncooperative patients, but it may be inaccurate even in very experienced hands. In general, tactile tensions are only useful for detecting large differences between two eyes.

## Infection Control in Clinical Tonometry

Many infectious agents, including the viruses responsible for acquired immunodeficiency syndrome (AIDS), hepatitis, and epidemic keratoconjunctivitis, can be recovered from tears. To prevent transfer of such agents, tonometers must be cleaned after each use:

□ The prism head of both the Goldmann-type tonometer and the Perkins tonometer should be cleaned immediately after use. The prisms should either be soaked in a 1:10 sodium hypochlorite solution or be thoroughly wiped with 70% ethanol. If a soaking solution is used, the prism should be rinsed and dried before reuse. If alcohol is employed, it should be allowed to evaporate, or the prism head should be dried before reuse, to prevent damage to the epithelium.

☐ The air-puff tonometer front surface should be wiped with alcohol between uses because tears from the patient may contaminate the instrument.

☐ The portable electronic applanation devices employ a disposable cover, which should be replaced immediately after each use.

☐ The Schiøtz tonometer requires disassembly to clean both the plunger and the footplate. Unless the plunger is clean (as opposed to sterile), the measurements may be falsely elevated because of increased friction between the plunger and the footplate. The inside of the footplate can be cleaned of tears and any tear film debris with a pipe cleaner. The same solutions used for cleaning prism heads may then be employed to sterilize the instrument.

For other tonometers, consult the manufacturer's recommendations.

Alm A, Weinreb RN, eds. *Uveoscleral Outflow: Biology and Clinical Aspects.* London: Mosby International; 1998.

# CHAPTER III

# Clinical Evaluation

## History and General Examination

Appropriate management of glaucoma depends on the clinician's ability to diagnose the specific form of glaucoma in a given patient, to determine the severity of the condition, and to detect progression in that patient's disease status. The most important aspects of the clinical evaluation of a glaucoma patient are discussed below.

### History

The history should include the following:

- The patient's current complaint
- Symptoms, onset, duration, severity, location
- Ocular history
- History of present illness
- Past ocular medical and surgical history
- General medical history
- Past systemic medical history (including medications and allergies)
- Review of systems
- Social history
- History of ethanol and tobacco
- Occupation, avocation, interests
- Family history

It is often useful to question the patient specifically regarding symptoms and conditions sometimes related to glaucoma, such as pain, redness, haloes, alteration of vision, or loss of vision. Similarly, the general medical history should include specific inquiry regarding diseases that may have ocular manifestations or may affect the patient's ability to tolerate medication. Such conditions include diabetes, cardiac and pulmonary disease, hypertension, shock, migraine and other neurologic diseases, and renal stones. In addition to identifying present medications and medication allergies, the clinician should take note of a history of corticosteroid use. See also BCSC Section 1, *Update on General Medicine,* for further discussion of these conditions and medications.

## Refraction

Neutralizing any refractive error is crucial for accurate perimetry, and the clinician should understand how the patient's refractive state affects the diagnosis. Hyperopic eyes are at increased risk of angle-closure glaucoma and generally have smaller discs. Myopia is associated with disc morphologies that can be clinically confused with glaucoma, and myopic eyes are at increased risk for pigment dispersion. Whether myopic eyes have increased risk of open-angle glaucoma remains a controversial issue.

## External Adnexae

Examination and assessment of the external ocular adnexae is useful in determining the presence of a variety of conditions associated with secondary glaucomas as well as external ocular manifestations of glaucoma therapy. The entities described below are discussed in greater depth and illustrated in other volumes of the BCSC series; consult the *Master Index*.

The glaucoma associated with *tuberous sclerosis (Bourneville syndrome),* may occur secondary to vitreous hemorrhage, anterior segment neovascularization, or retinal detachment. Typical external and cutaneous signs of tuberous sclerosis include a hypopigmented lesion termed the "ash-leaf" sign and a red-brown papular rash (adenoma sebaceum) that is often found on the face and chin.

Glaucoma is commonly associated with *neurofibromatosis (von Recklinghausen disease),* likely secondary to developmental abnormalities of the anterior chamber angle. Subcutaneous plexiform neuromas are a hallmark of the type 1 variant of neurofibromatosis. When found in the upper eyelid, the plexiform neuroma can produce a classic S-shaped upper eyelid deformity strongly associated with risk of glaucoma.

In *juvenile xanthogranuloma* yellow and/or orange papules are commonly found on the skin of the head and neck. Secondary glaucoma may cause acute pain and photophobia and ultimately significant visual loss. *Oculodermal melanocytosis (nevus of Ota)* presents with the key finding of hyperpigmentation of periocular skin. Intraocular pigmentation is also increased, which contributes to a higher incidence of glaucoma and may possibly increase the risk of malignant melanoma. *Axenfeld-Rieger syndrome,* an autosomal dominant disorder with variable penetrance, is associated with microdontia (small, peglike incisors), hypodontia (decreased number of teeth), and anodontia (focal absence of teeth). Maxillary hypoplasia may also be present. Glaucoma occurs in 50% of cases in late childhood or adulthood.

A number of entities are associated with signs of increased episcleral venous pressure. The presence of a facial cutaneous angioma (nevus flammeus, or a port-wine stain) can indicate *encephalofacial angiomatosis (Sturge-Weber syndrome).* Hemifacial hypertrophy may also be observed. The cutaneous hemangiomas of the *Klippel-Trénaunay-Weber syndrome* extend over an affected, secondarily hypertrophied limb and may also involve the face.

*Orbital varices* are associated with secondary glaucoma. Intermittent unilateral proptosis and dilated eyelid veins are key external signs of orbital varices. Carotid cavernous, dural cavernous, and other *arteriovenous fistulae* can produce orbital bruits, restricted ocular motility, proptosis, and pulsating exophthalmos. *Superior vena cava syndrome* can cause proptosis and facial and eyelid edema, as well as conjunctival chemosis. *Thyroid ophthalmopathy* and its associated glaucoma are associated with exophthalmos, eyelid retraction, and motility disorders.

Use of topical prostaglandin analogues may result in trichiasis, distichiasis, and growth of facial hair around the eyes as well as increased skin pigmentation involving the eyelids. Use of glaucoma hypotensive agents may also result in an allergic contact dermatitis. Chapter VII, Medical Management of Glaucoma, discusses these agents in detail.

## Pupils

Pupil size may be affected by glaucoma therapy, and pupillary responses are one measure of compliance in patients who are on miotic therapy. Testing for a relative afferent pupillary defect may detect asymmetric optic nerve damage, a common and important finding in glaucoma. Corectopia, ectropion uveae, and pupillary abnormalities may also be observed in some forms of glaucoma. In some clinical situations it is not possible to assess the pupils objectively for the presence of a relative afferent defect. Under those circumstances it can be useful to ask the patient to make a subjective comparison between the eyes of the perceived brightness of a test light.

## Biomicroscopy

Biomicroscopy of the anterior segment is performed for signs of underlying or associated ocular disease. BCSC Section 8, *External Disease and Cornea,* discusses slit-lamp technique and the examination of the external eye in greater depth.

**Conjunctiva** Eyes with acutely elevated IOP may show conjunctival vasodilation. The chronic elevation of IOP that can occur in arteriovenous fistulae may produce massive episcleral venous dilation. Chronic use of sympathomimetic drops may also cause conjunctival injection, and chronic use of epinephrine derivatives may result in black adrenochrome deposits in the conjunctiva (see Figure VII-1). The use of topical antiglaucoma medication can also cause decreased tear production, allergic and hypersensitivity reactions (papillary and follicular conjunctivitis), foreshortening of the conjunctival fornices, and scarring. The presence or absence of any filtering bleb should be noted. If a bleb is present, its size, height, degree of vascularization, and integrity should be noted.

**Episclera and sclera** Dilation of the episcleral vessels may indicate elevated episcleral venous pressure, a finding that can be seen in the secondary glaucomas associated with Sturge-Weber syndrome or in arteriovenous fistulae. Sentinel vessels may be seen in eyes harboring an intraocular tumor. Any thinning or staphylomatous areas should be noted.

**Cornea** Enlargement of the cornea associated with breaks in Descemet's membrane (Haab's striae) is commonly found in developmental glaucoma patients. Glaucomas associated with other anterior segment anomalies are described below. Punctate epithelial defects, especially in the inferonasal interpalpebral region, are often indicative of medication toxicity. Microcystic epithelial edema is commonly associated with elevated IOP, particularly when the pressure rise is acute. Corneal endothelial abnormalities can be important clues to the presence of an underlying associated secondary glaucoma, for example:

- Krukenberg spindle in pigmentary glaucoma
- Deposition of exfoliation material in exfoliation syndrome
- Keratic precipitates in uveitic glaucoma
- Guttae in Fuchs endothelial dystrophy
- Irregular and vesicular lesions in posterior polymorphous dystrophy
- A "beaten bronze" appearance in the iridocorneal endothelial syndrome

An anteriorly displaced Schwalbe's line is found in Axenfeld-Rieger syndrome. The presence of traumatic or surgical corneal scars should be noted. The assessment of corneal thickness can also be important in some patients whose IOP may be inconsistent with their clinical examination or when measurement error by applanation tonometry is suspected.

**Anterior chamber**  To estimate the width of the chamber angle, the examiner directs a narrow slit beam at an angle of 60° onto the cornea just anterior to the limbus (Van Herick method). If the distance from the anterior iris surface to the posterior surface of the cornea is less than one fourth the thickness of the cornea, the angle may be narrow. This test should alert the examiner to narrow angles, but it is not a substitute for gonioscopy, which is discussed in detail below (Figs III-1, III-2, Table III-1).

The uniformity of depth of the anterior chamber should be noted. Iris bombé can result in an anterior chamber that is deep centrally and shallow or flat peripherally. Iris masses can produce an irregular iris surface contour and nonuniformity in anterior chamber depth. In many circumstances, especially in the assessment of narrow-angle glaucoma, comparison of chamber depth between eyes is of significant value. The presence of inflammatory cells, red cells, ghost cells, fibrin, vitreous,

TABLE III-1

GONIOSCOPIC EXAMINATION

| TISSUE | FEATURES |
| --- | --- |
| Posterior cornea | Pigmentation, guttata |
| Schwalbe's line | Thickening, anterior displacement |
| Trabecular meshwork | Pigmentation, peripheral anterior synechiae (PAS), inflammatory or neovascular membranes, keratic precipitates |
| Scleral spur | Iris processes, presence or absence |
| Ciliary body band | Width, regularity, cyclodialysis cleft |
| Iris | Contour, rubeosis, atrophy, cysts, iridodonesis |
| Pupil and lens | Exfoliation syndrome, posterior synechiae, position and regularity, sphincter rupture, ectropion uveae |
| Zonular fibers | Pigmentation, rupture |

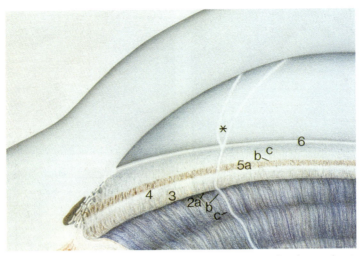

FIG III-1—Gonioscopic appearance of a normal anterior chamber angle. *2,* Peripheral iris: *a,* insertion; *b,* curvature; *c,* angular approach. *3,* Ciliary body band. *4,* Scleral spur. *5,* Trabecular meshwork: *a,* posterior; *b,* mid; *c,* anterior. *6,* Schwalbe's line. *Asterisk,* Corneal optical wedge.

or other findings should be noted. The degree of inflammation (flare and cell) should be determined prior to instillation of eyedrops.

***Iris*** Examination should be performed prior to dilation. Heterochromia, iris atrophy, transillumination defects, ectropion uveae, corectopia, nevi, nodules, and exfoliative material should be noted. Early stages of neovascularization of the anterior segment may appear as either fine tufts around the pupillary margin or as a fine network of vessels on the surface of the iris. The iris should also be examined for evidence of trauma, such as sphincter tears or iridodonesis. The degree of baseline iris pigmentation should be noted, especially in patients being considered for treatment with a prostaglandin analogue.

***Lens*** The lens is generally best examined after dilation. Exfoliative material, phacodonesis, subluxation, and dislocation should be noted along with lens size, shape, and clarity. A posterior subcapsular cataract may be indicative of chronic corticosteroid use. An intraocular foreign body with siderosis and glaucoma may also result in characteristic lens changes. The presence, type, and position of an intraocular lens should be recorded along with the status of the posterior capsule.

***Fundus*** Careful assessment of the optic disc is an essential part of the clinical examination for glaucoma, and this is covered in detail below. In addition, fundus examination may reveal posterior segment pathology such as hemorrhages, effusions, masses, inflammatory lesions, retinovascular occlusions, diabetic retinopathy, or retinal detachments that can be associated with the glaucomas. Funduscopy is best performed with a dilated pupil.

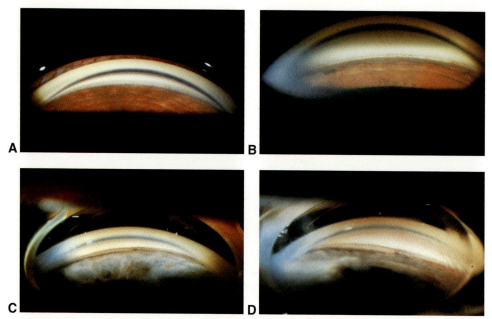

FIG III-2—*A*, Normal open angle. Gonioscopic photograph shows trace pigmentation of the posterior trabecular meshwork and normal insertion of the iris into a narrow ciliary body band. The Goldmann lens was used. *B*, Normal open angle. This gonioscopic view using the Goldmann lens shows mild pigmentation of the posterior trabecular meshwork. A wide ciliary body band with posterior insertion of the iris can also be seen. *C*, Narrow angle. This gonioscopic view using the Zeiss lens without indentation shows pigment in inferior angle but poor visualization of angle anatomy. *D*, Narrow angle. Gonioscopy with a Zeiss lens with indentation shows peripheral anterior synechiae in the posterior trabecular meshwork. Pigment deposits on Schwalbe's line can also be seen. This is the same angle as shown in *C*. (Photographs courtesy of Elizabeth A. Hodapp, MD.)

## Gonioscopy

Gonioscopy is an essential diagnostic tool in glaucoma. Gonioscopic expertise is also crucial for accurate glaucoma treatment in the angle (e.g., laser trabeculoplasty). Gonioscopy should be performed as part of the initial evaluation of all patients able to cooperate with the test and should be repeated periodically. Figures III-1 and III-2 give schematic and clinical views of the angle as seen with gonioscopy.

Under normal conditions the anterior chamber angle cannot be viewed directly through the cornea, because light coming from the angle undergoes total internal reflection at the tear film–air interface. Because the index of refraction of glass or plastic is similar to that of the cornea and tears, gonioscopy eliminates this interface and replaces it with a new lens–air interface set at a different angle to the emerging rays. Depending on the type of lens employed, the angle can be examined with a direct system (e.g., Koeppe) or a mirrored indirect (Goldmann-type or Zeiss-type) system (Fig III-3).

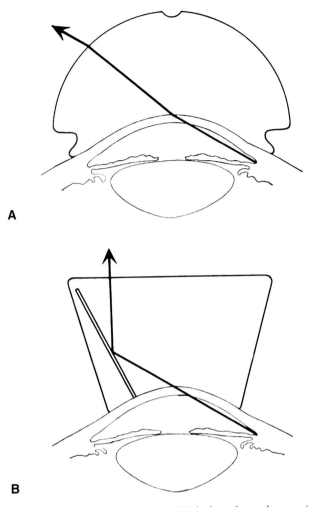

**A**

**B**

FIG III-3—*A*, Direct gonioscopy. Diagram of rays of light from the angle emerging through a Koeppe lens. *B*, Indirect gonioscopy. Diagram of rays of light emerging through a Goldmann lens. (Reproduced with permission from Kolker AE, Hetherington J, eds. *Becker-Shaffer's Diagnosis and Therapy of the Glaucomas.* 5th ed. St Louis: Mosby; 1983.)

## Indirect Gonioscopy

Indirect gonioscopy can be performed rapidly and easily. A *goniolens* containing a mirror or mirrors yields an inverted and slightly foreshortened image of the opposite angle. Although the image is inverted with an indirect goniolens, the right–left orientation of a horizontal mirror and the up–down orientation of a vertical mirror remain unchanged. The foreshortening, combined with the upright position of the patient, makes the angle appear a little shallower than it does with direct gonioscopy systems. Indirect goniolenses are used in conjunction with standard slit lamps, which provide magnification and illumination. They may also be used in the operating room in conjunction with a surgical microscope.

Examining the deepest aspect of a narrow angle with an indirect goniolens may be difficult. Visibility can be improved by tilting the mirror toward the angle in question or rotating the eye toward the viewing mirror, using a fixation light before the fellow eye, or asking the patient to look toward the mirror the examiner is attempting to view the angle through.

The *Goldmann-type* goniolens requires a viscous fluid such as methylcellulose for optical coupling with the cornea. In lenses with only one mirror, the lens must be rotated to view the entire angle. Posterior pressure on the lens, especially if it is tilted, indents the sclera and may falsely narrow the angle. The combination of lens manipulation and the use of viscous coupling fluid often temporarily reduces the clarity of the cornea and may make subsequent fundus examination, visual field testing, and photography more difficult.

The *Zeiss-type* lens and similar goniolenses with a smaller area of contact than the Goldmann-type lens have about the same radius of curvature as the cornea and are optically coupled by the patient's tears. Since the Zeiss-type lens has four mirrors, the entire angle is visible without rotation during examination. The diameter of the lens is smaller than the diameter of the cornea, and pressure on the cornea may distort the chamber angle. The examiner can detect this pressure by noting the induced folds in Descemet's membrane. Although pressure may falsely open the angle, the technique of indentation or compression (indentation gonioscopy) is useful, and sometimes essential, in distinguishing iridocorneal apposition from synechial closure. Because of the small diameter of the Zeiss-type lens, pressure pushes aqueous humor from the center of the anterior chamber into the periphery. This action displaces iris tissue that is touching the trabecular meshwork, but it cannot displace peripheral anterior synechiae (PAS) (Fig III-4).

## Direct Gonioscopy

Direct gonioscopy is performed with a binocular microscope, a fiberoptic illuminator or slit-pen light, and a direct goniolens such as the Koeppe, Barkan, Wurst, or Richardson. The *Koeppe lens* has a space filled with a saline solution or gonioscopic gel to couple the lens optically to the cornea. This system requires the patient to be supine. Koeppe-type lenses provide a direct panoramic view of the angle. The examiner is able to vary the direction of the light and the direction of viewing, which is helpful in identifying landmarks and examining narrow angles. Koeppe gonioscopy is particularly useful for comparing angles or portions of angles; for example, to diagnose angle recession.

The Koeppe lens and other direct lenses find their greatest utility in the operating room for examinations and for surgical procedures of the angle such as goniotomy. Koeppe-type lenses are also quite useful in performing funduscopy. When used with a direct ophthalmoscope and high-plus-power lens, they can provide a good view of the fundus even through a very small pupil. These lenses are especially helpful in individuals with nystagmus or irregular corneas. Inconvenience is the major disadvantage of the direct gonioscopy systems.

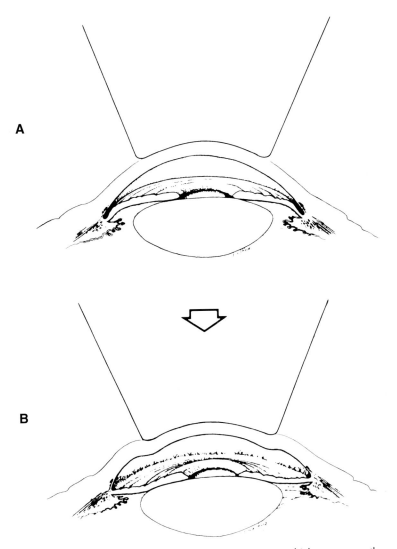

**A**

**B**

FIG III-4—Pressure gonioscopy. Demonstration of the manner in which pressure on the cornea displaces iris to widen a narrow or closed anterior chamber angle. This maneuver exposes additional anatomical landmarks and is useful in determining the presence or absence of PAS. Synechiae, if present, can sometimes be separated. *A,* Without pressure. *B,* With pressure. (Reproduced with permission from Hoskins HD Jr, Kass MA, eds. *Becker-Shaffer's Diagnosis and Therapy of the Glaucomas.* 6th ed. St Louis: Mosby; 1989.)

## Gonioscopic Assessment and Classification

In performing both direct and indirect gonioscopy, the clinician must recognize the angle landmarks. The scleral spur and Schwalbe's line are the most consistent and helpful of these for orientation. With slit-lamp gonioscopy the examiner can locate Schwalbe's line at the termination of the corneal light wedge. Using a narrow slit beam and sharp focus, the examiner sees two linear reflections, one from the external surface of the cornea and its junction with the sclera, the other from the internal surface of the cornea. The two reflections meet at Schwalbe's line (see Figure III-1). The scleral spur is a thin, pale stripe between the ciliary face and the pigmented zone of the trabecular meshwork. The inferior portion of the angle is generally wider and is the easiest place in which to locate the landmarks. After verifying the landmarks, the clinician should examine the entire angle in an orderly manner (see Table III-1).

Proper management of glaucoma requires that the clinician determine not only whether the angle is open or closed, but also whether or not other pathologic findings such as angle recession or low PAS are present. In angle closure the peripheral iris obstructs the trabecular meshwork; i.e., the meshwork is not visible on gonioscopy. The width of the angle is determined by the site of insertion of the iris on the ciliary face, the convexity of the iris, and the prominence of the peripheral iris roll. In many cases the angle appears open but very narrow. It is often difficult to distinguish a narrow but open angle from an angle with partial closure; indentation gonioscopy is useful in this situation (see Figure III-2).

The best method for describing the angle is a description or drawing of the iris contour, the location of the iris insertion, and the angle between the iris and the trabecular meshwork. A variety of gonioscopic grading systems have been developed. All grading systems serve to facilitate standardized description of angle structures and to abbreviate their description. Thus, it should be kept in mind that by abbreviation, some details may be eliminated. The most commonly used gonioscopic grading systems are the Shaffer and Spaeth systems. A clinician who uses a grading system must specify which system is being used.

The *Shaffer system* describes the angle between the trabecular meshwork and the iris as follows:

☐ *Grade IV:* The angle between the iris and the surface of the trabecular meshwork is 45°.

☐ *Grade III:* The angle between the iris and the surface of the trabecular meshwork is greater than 20° but less than 45°.

☐ *Grade II:* The angle between the iris and the surface of the trabecular meshwork is 20°. Angle closure possible.

☐ *Grade I:* The angle between the iris and the surface of the trabecular meshwork is 10°. Angle closure probable in time.

☐ *Slit:* The angle between the iris and the surface of the trabecular meshwork is less than 10°. Angle closure very likely.

☐ *O:* The iris is against the trabecular meshwork. Angle closure is present.

The *Spaeth gonioscopic grading system* expands this system to include a description of the peripheral iris contour, the insertion of the iris root, and the effects of indentation gonioscopy on the angle configuration (Fig III-5).

Ordinarily, Schlemm's canal is invisible by gonioscopy. Occasionally during gonioscopy in normal eyes, blood refluxes into Schlemm's canal where it is seen as a faint red line in the posterior portion of the trabecular meshwork. Blood enters Schlemm's canal when episcleral venous pressure exceeds IOP, most commonly because of compression of the episcleral veins by the lip of the goniolens. Pathological causes include hypotony and elevated episcleral venous pressure, as in carotid cavernous fistula or Sturge-Weber syndrome.

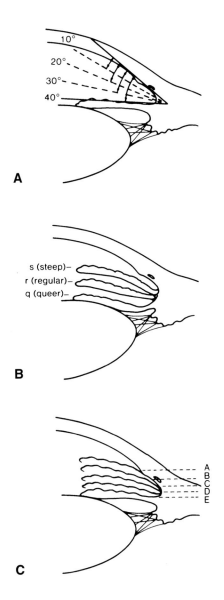

FIG III-5—Spaeth's gonioscopic classification of the anterior chamber angle, based on three variables: *A*, angular width of the angle recess; *B*, configuration of the peripheral iris; and *C*, apparent insertion of the iris root. (Reproduced with permission from Shields MB. *Textbook of Glaucoma*. 3rd ed. Baltimore: Williams & Wilkins; 1992.)

Normal blood vessels in the angle include radial iris vessels, portions of the arterial circle of the ciliary body, and vertical branches of the anterior ciliary arteries. Normal vessels are oriented either radially along the iris or circumferentially (in a serpentine manner) in the ciliary body face. Vessels that cross the scleral spur to reach the trabecular meshwork are usually abnormal (Fig III-6). The vessels seen in

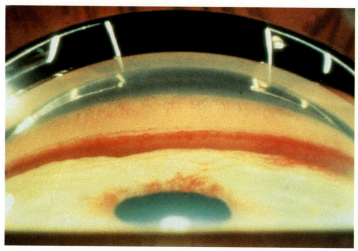

FIG III-6—Goniophoto of an eye with neovascularization of the angle. (Photograph courtesy of Tom Richardson, MD.)

Fuchs heterochromic iridocyclitis are fine, branching, unsheathed, and meandering. Patients with neovascular glaucoma have trunklike vessels crossing the ciliary body and scleral spur and arborizing over the trabecular meshwork. Contraction of the myofibroblasts accompanying these vessels leads to PAS formation.

It is important to distinguish PAS from iris processes (uveal meshwork), which are open and lacy and follow the normal curve of the angle. The angle structures are visible in the open spaces between the processes. Synechiae are more solid or sheet-like (Fig III-7). They are composed of iris stroma and obliterate the angle recess.

*Pigmentation of the trabecular meshwork* increases with age, and it is more marked in individuals with darkly pigmented irides. Pigmentation can be segmental and is usually most marked in the inferior angle. The pigmentation pattern of an individual angle is dynamic over time, especially in conditions such as pigment dispersion syndrome. Heavy pigmentation of the trabecular meshwork should suggest pigment dispersion or exfoliation syndrome. Other conditions that cause increased anterior chamber angle pigmentation include malignant melanoma, trauma, surgery, inflammation, and hyphema. Some of these conditions are associated with pigmentation anterior to Schwalbe's line.

*Posttraumatic angle recession* may be associated with monocular open-angle glaucoma. The gonioscopic criteria for diagnosing angle recession include

□ An abnormally wide ciliary body band

□ Increased prominence of the sclera spur

□ Torn iris processes

□ Sclera visible through disrupted ciliary body tissue

□ Marked variation of ciliary face width and angle depth in different quadrants of the same eye

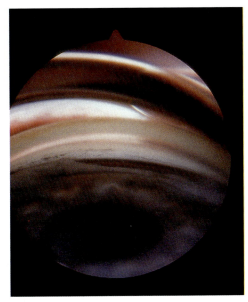

FIG III-7—Goniophoto showing both an area of sheetlike PAS (left) and open angle (right).

In evaluating for angle recession it is helpful to compare one portion of the angle to other areas in the same eye or to the same area in the fellow eye.

Figure III-8 illustrates the variety of gonioscopic findings caused by blunt trauma. If the ciliary body separates from the scleral spur (cyclodialysis), it will appear gonioscopically as a deep angle recess with a gap between the sclera and the ciliary body. Detection of a very small cleft may require ultrasound biomicroscopy. Other findings that may be visible gonioscopically are

- Microhyphema or hypopyon
- Retained anterior chamber foreign body
- Iridodialysis
- Angle precipitates suggestive of glaucomatocyclitic crisis
- Pigmentation of the lens equator
- Other peripheral lens abnormalities
- Ciliary body tumors

Campbell DG. A comparison of diagnostic techniques in angle-closure glaucoma. *Am J Ophthalmol.* 1979;88:197–204.

Fellman RL, Spaeth GL, Starita RJ. Gonioscopy: key to successful management of glaucoma. In: *Focal Points: Clinical Modules for Ophthalmologists.* San Francisco: American Academy of Ophthalmology; 1984: vol 2, no 7.

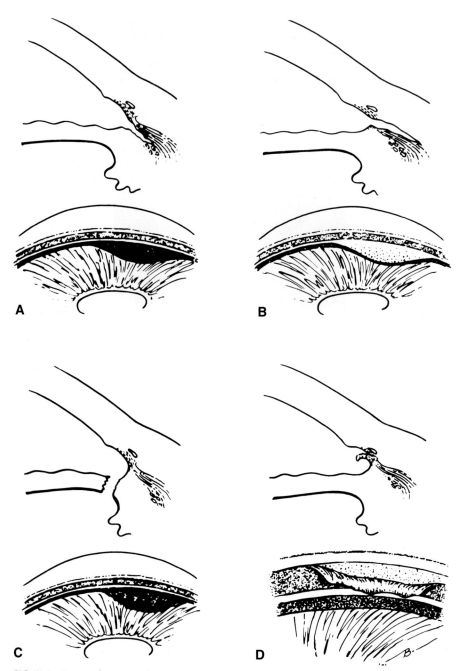

FIG III-8—Forms of anterior chamber angle injury associated with blunt trauma, showing cross-sectional and corresponding gonioscopic appearance. *A*, Angle recession (tear between longitudinal and circular muscles of ciliary body). *B*, Cyclodialysis (separation of ciliary body from scleral spur) with widening of suprachoroidal space. *C*, Iridodialysis (tear in root of iris). *D*, Trabecular damage (tear in anterior portion of meshwork, creating a flap that is hinged at the scleral spur). (Reproduced with permission from Shields MB. *Textbook of Glaucoma*. 3rd ed. Baltimore: Williams & Wilkins; 1992.)

## The Optic Nerve

The entire visual pathway is described and illustrated in BCSC Section 5, *Neuro-Ophthalmology*. For further discussion of retinal involvement in the visual process, see Section 12, *Retina and Vitreous*.

### Anatomy and Pathology

The optic nerve head is composed of neural tissue, glial tissue, extracellular matrix, and blood vessels. The human optic nerve consists of approximately 1.2 million axons, although there is significant individual variability. The cell bodies of these axons lie in the ganglion cell layer of the retina. The axons are separated into fascicles, with the intervening spaces occupied by astrocytes. The average diameter of the intraocular portion of the nerve is 1.5 mm.

In primates two main subpopulations of retinal ganglion cells are currently recognized: *magnocellular neurons (M cells)* and *parvocellular neurons (P cells)*. Approximately 10% of retinal ganglion cells are large M cells. They have large-diameter axons, synapse in the magnocellular layer of the lateral geniculate body, and are sensitive to luminance changes in dim illumination (scotopic conditions). The smaller P cells account for approximately 90% of all ganglion cells. In comparison to the M cells, the P cells have smaller-diameter axons, smaller receptive fields, and slower conduction velocity. They synapse in the parvocellular layers of the lateral geniculate body. P cells subserve color vision, are most active under higher luminance conditions, and discriminate fine detail.

The distribution of nerve fibers as they enter the optic nerve head is shown in Figure III-9. The arcuate nerve fibers entering the superior and inferior poles of the disc seem to be more susceptible to glaucomatous damage. This susceptibility explains the frequent occurrence of arcuate nerve fiber bundle visual field defects in glaucoma. The arrangement of the axons in the optic nerve head and their differential susceptibility to damage determines the patterns of visual field loss seen in glaucoma, which are described and illustrated later in this chapter.

The optic nerve head can be divided into four layers (Fig III-10):

□ Nerve fiber

□ Prelaminar

□ Laminar

□ Retrolaminar

The most superficial, the *nerve fiber layer*, can be viewed with the ophthalmoscope using the red-free (green) filter (red-free ophthalmoscopy). This tissue is supported by astrocytes and receives its vascular supply predominantly from the central retinal artery. The short posterior ciliary artery circulation may contribute to the temporal nerve fiber layer vascular supply.

The second layer of the nerve head, the *prelaminar layer*, is seen clinically only in the area of the central optic cup, the depression in the center of the optic disc. This layer receives the axons of the optic nerve as they angle posteriorly from the plane of the retina to the optic nerve. The blood supply of the prelaminar layer comes primarily from the short posterior ciliary arteries.

The third layer, the *laminar layer*, is a fenestrated area of connective tissue termed the *lamina cribrosa*, through which nerve fibers exit from the eye. Histologically, the *lamina cribrosa* appears as a series of approximately 10 stacked plates of fenestrated connective tissue whose septae contain small blood vessels. The gray

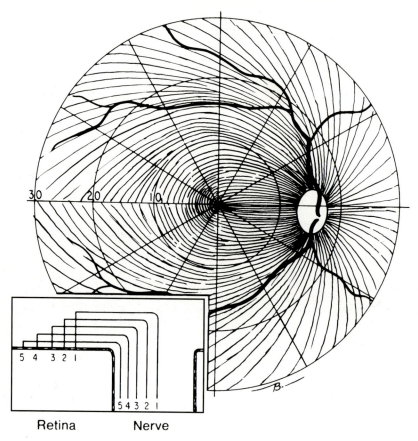

Retina       Nerve

FIG III-9—Anatomy of retinal nerve fiber distribution. Inset depicts cross-sectional view of axonal arrangement. Peripheral fibers run closer to choroid and exit in periphery of optic nerve, while fibers originating closer to the nerve head are situated closer to the vitreous and occupy a more central portion of the nerve. (Reproduced with permission from Shields MB. *Textbook of Glaucoma*. 3rd ed. Baltimore: Williams & Wilkins; 1992.)

dots that can sometimes be seen ophthalmoscopically in the depths of the optic cup are the superficial openings of the lamina. In hyperopic eyes the lamina cribrosa is approximately 0.7 mm posterior to the retinal plane, whereas in myopic eyes it is half that distance. The vascular supply to the laminar region also comes primarily from the short posterior ciliary arteries (Fig III-11).

The optic nerve branches of the short posterior ciliary artery differ from its branches in the choriocapillaris in three ways: they are surrounded by pericytes, they lack fenestrations, and they have tight junctions. That is, they resemble central nervous system and retinal capillaries. Under normal circumstances, the optic nerve head branches of the short posterior ciliary artery autoregulate. In contrast, the choroidal circulation appears to lack the ability to autoregulate. Various studies suggest that autoregulatory dysfunction of the blood supply to the nerve is present in some forms of glaucoma.

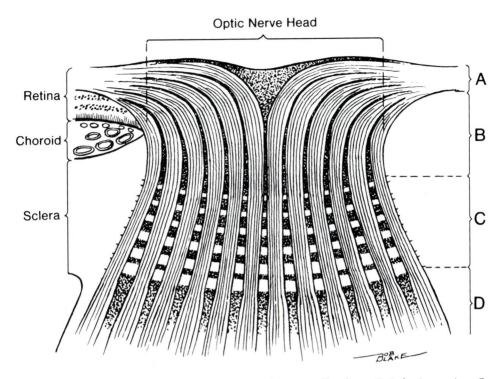

FIG III-10—Divisions of the optic nerve head. *A,* Surface nerve fiber layer. *B,* Prelaminar region. *C,* Lamina cribrosa region. *D,* Retrolaminar region. (Reproduced with permission from Shields MB. *Textbook of Glaucoma.* 3rd ed. Baltimore: Williams & Wilkins; 1992.)

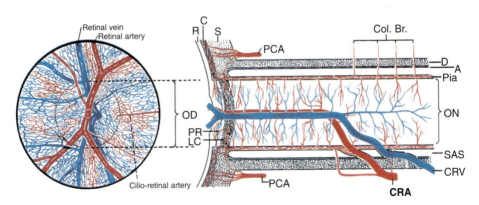

FIG III-11—Diagrammatic representation of blood supply of the optic nerve head and intraorbital optic nerve. *A,* Arachnoid; *C,* Choroid; *CRA,* Central retinal artery; *Col Br,* Collateral branches; *CRV,* Central retinal vein; *D,* Dura; *LC,* Lamina cribrosa; *OD,* Optic disc; *ON,* Optic nerve; *PCA,* Posterior ciliary arteries; *PR,* Prelaminar region; *R,* Retina; *S,* Sclera; *SAS,* Subarachnoid space. (Reproduced by permission from Hayreh SS. Anatomy and physiology of the optic nerve head. *Trans Am Acad Ophthalmol Otolaryngol.* 1974;78:240–254.)

The *retrolaminar portion* of the optic nerve extends posteriorly from the lamina cribrosa and thus lies outside the globe. The addition of the myelin sheath produced by oligodendrocytes doubles the diameter of the nerve at this point. The vascular supply to the retrolaminar nerve comes from branches of the meningeal arteries and centrifugal branches of the central retinal artery.

***Glaucomatous cupping***   On a histologic level early glaucomatous cupping consists of loss of axons, blood vessels, and glial cells. The loss of tissue seems to start at the level of the lamina cribrosa and is associated with compaction and fusion of the laminar plates. It is most pronounced at the superior and inferior poles of the disc. Disc changes may precede detectable visual field loss.

Tissue destruction in more advanced glaucoma extends behind the cribriform plate, and the lamina bows backward. The optic nerve head takes on an excavated and undermined appearance that has been likened to a bean pot.

Glaucomatous cupping in infants and children is accompanied by an expansion of the entire scleral ring, which may explain why cupping seems to occur earlier in children and why reversibility of cupping is more prominent with successful treatment in these cases. Cupping may be reversed in adults as well, but such reversal is less frequent and more subtle.

## Theories of Glaucomatous Damage

Elevated IOP is one etiological factor in glaucomatous optic neuropathy. Unilateral secondary glaucoma, experimentally induced glaucoma, and observations of the effect of lowering IOP in patients with glaucoma all point to this conclusion. But it is also clear that factors other than pressure contribute to a given individual's susceptibility to glaucomatous damage.

It has become common to discuss the theories of glaucomatous damage as if they fell into two categories, mechanical and ischemic. The *mechanical theory* stresses the importance of direct compression of the optic nerve fibers against the lamina cribrosa with interruption of axoplasmic flow, while the *ischemic theory* stresses the possible effects of IOP on the blood supply to the nerve.

A recent theory of particular interest suggests that a disturbance of *autoregulation* may contribute to nerve damage. The optic nerve vessels normally increase or decrease their tone to maintain a constant blood flow independent of IOP. A disturbance in autoregulation may cause the blood flow in the optic nerve to decrease with increased IOP or to exhibit vasospasm, even at normal IOP. Such hypothetical derangement could be related to abnormal vessels or to circulating vasoactive substances, for example.

Current thinking regarding glaucomatous damage recognizes that a variety of both vascular and mechanical factors probably combine to damage the optic nerve at the lamina. The glaucomas are likely a heterogeneous family of disorders, and the ganglion cell death seen in glaucomatous optic neuropathy may be mediated by many factors. Active investigations continue to examine the role of processes such as excitotoxicity, apoptosis, neurotrophin deprivation, ischemia, molecular biologic abnormalities, and autoimmunity in leading to ganglion cell death.

## Examination of the Optic Nerve Head

The optic disc can be examined clinically with a direct ophthalmoscope, an indirect ophthalmoscope, or a slit-lamp biomicroscope using a posterior pole lens. The instrument most commonly used by nonophthalmologists to examine the optic disc is the *direct ophthalmoscope,* which is simple to learn and inexpensive in comparison to other instruments. The direct ophthalmoscope can successfully be employed to provide a view of the optic disc through a small pupil. In addition, when used with a red-free filter, it provides a view of the nerve fiber layer of the posterior pole. However, the direct ophthalmoscope does not provide sufficient stereoscopic detail to detect subtle changes in optic disc topography.

The *indirect ophthalmoscope* is used for examining the optic disc in young children, uncooperative patients, highly myopic individuals, and individuals with substantial opacities of the media. The view obtained usually suggests both less cupping and less pallor than do slit-lamp methods, and the magnification is often inadequate for detecting subtle or localized details important in the evaluation of glaucoma. Thus, the indirect ophthalmoscope is not recommended for routine use in examining the optic disc.

The best method of examination for the diagnosis of glaucoma is the *slit lamp* combined with a Hruby lens; a posterior pole contact lens; or a 60-, 78-, or 90-diopter lens. The slit beam, rather than diffuse illumination, is useful for determining subtle changes in the contour of the nerve head. This system provides high magnification, excellent illumination, and a stereoscopic view of the disc. However, slit-lamp techniques require significant patient cooperation and moderate pupil size for adequate visibility of the disc.

## Clinical Evaluation of the Optic Nerve Head

The *optic disc* is usually round or slightly oval in shape, and it contains a central *cup.* The tissue between the cup and the disc margin is called the *neural rim* or *neuroretinal rim.* The rim in normal patients has a relatively uniform width and a color that ranges from orange to pink.

The size of the physiologic cup is genetically determined and is related to the size of the disc. For a given number of nerve fibers, the larger the overall disc area, the larger the cup. Cup/disc ratio may increase slightly with age. Nonglaucomatous black individuals have, on the average, larger disc areas and larger cup/disc ratios than do whites, although a substantial overlap exists. Myopes have larger eyes and larger discs and cups than do emmetropes and hyperopes.

Differentiating physiologic or normal cupping from acquired *glaucomatous cupping* of the optic disc can be difficult. The early changes of glaucomatous *optic neuropathy* are very subtle (Table III-2):

□ Generalized enlargement of the cup

□ Focal enlargement of the cup

□ Superficial splinter hemorrhage

□ Loss of nerve fiber layer

□ Translucency of the neuroretinal rim

□ Development of vessel overpass

□ Asymmetry of cupping between the patient's two eyes

TABLE III-2

OPHTHALMOSCOPIC SIGNS OF GLAUCOMA

| GENERALIZED | FOCAL | LESS SPECIFIC |
|---|---|---|
| Large optic cup | Narrowing (notching) of the rim | Exposed lamina cribrosa |
| Asymmetry of the cups | Vertical elongation of the cup | Nasal displacement of vessels |
| Progressive enlargement of the cup | Cupping to the rim margin | Baring of circumlinear vessels |
| | Regional pallor | Peripapillary crescent |
| | Splinter hemorrhage | |
| | Nerve fiber layer loss | |

Generalized enlargement of the cup may be the earliest change detected in glaucoma. This enlargement can be difficult to appreciate unless previous photographs or diagrams are available. It is useful to compare one eye to the fellow eye, because disc asymmetry is unusual in normal individuals (Fig III-12). Examination of other family members may clarify whether a large cup is inherited or acquired.

Focal enlargement of the cup appears as localized notching or narrowing of the rim. Deep localized notching where the lamina cribrosa is visible at the disc margin is sometimes termed an *acquired optic disc pit formation*. If notching or acquired pit formation occurs at either (or both) the superior or inferior pole of the disc, the cup becomes vertically oval (Fig III-13).

Splinter hemorrhage usually appears as a linear red streak on or near the disc surface (Fig III-I4). The hemorrhage clears over several weeks to months but is often followed by localized notching and pallor of the rim and visual field loss. Some glaucoma patients have repeated episodes of optic disc hemorrhage, while others have none. Individuals with normal-tension glaucoma are particularly likely to have disc

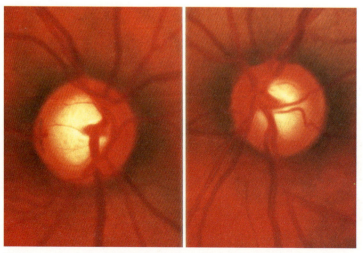

FIG III-12—Asymmetry of optic discs. The right disc *(left photograph)* is distinctly more cupped than the left disc *(right photograph)*.

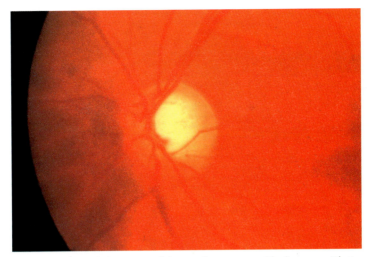

FIG III-13—Vertical elongation of the cup in a person with glaucoma. (Photograph courtesy of Elizabeth A. Hodapp, MD.)

hemorrhages. Optic disc hemorrhage is an important prognostic sign for the development or progression of visual field loss. Although some patients may experience disc hemorrhage without apparent exacerbation of disc damage, any patient with an optic disc hemorrhage requires detailed evaluation and follow-up.

Glaucomatous optic atrophy is associated with loss of axons in the nerve fiber layer. In the normal eye the nerve fiber layer may best be visualized with red-free

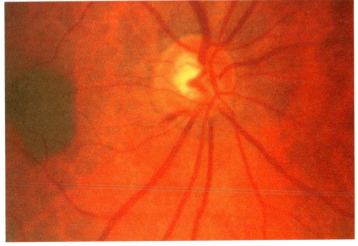

FIG III-14—Splinter hemorrhage of optic disc at 7 o'clock. (Photograph courtesy of Elizabeth A. Hodapp, MD.)

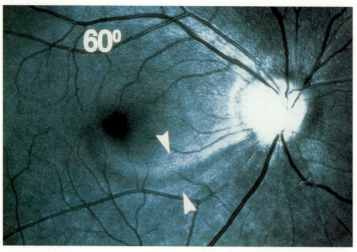

FIG III-15—Nerve fiber layer photograph shows a nerve fiber bundle defect (arrowheads).

illumination; it appears as a pattern of striations that radiate toward the optic disc. With the development of glaucoma, the nerve fiber layer thins and becomes less visible. The loss may be diffuse (generalized) or localized to specific bundles (Fig III-15). The nerve fiber layer can be seen most clearly in high-contrast black-and-white photographs, and experienced observers can recognize even early disease if good-quality photographs are available.

In the early stages of nerve fiber loss, often before enlargement of the cup, existing neuroretinal rim tissue can be observed to become more translucent. The clinician can best observe this rim translucency by using a lens at the slit-lamp biomicroscope, employing a thin slit beam and confining the beam to the disc surface.

As the nerve fiber loss continues, the cup may begin to enlarge by progressive posterior collapse and compaction of the remaining viable nerve fibers. In circumstances where the neuroretinal tissue, but not the overlying nerve head vasculature, has collapsed, vessel overpass can often be observed. The blood vessels overlying the collapsed neural rim tissue appear like a highway overpass suspended over, but not in contact with, the underlying tissue.

Peripapillary atrophy is often observed in glaucomatous eyes. It is seen with greater frequency and is more extensive in eyes with glaucoma than in unaffected eyes. The location of the atrophy often correlates with the position of visual field defects. Other less specific signs of glaucomatous damage include nasal displacement of the vessels, narrowing of peripapillary retinal vessels, and baring of the circumlinear vessels. With advanced damage the cup becomes pale and markedly excavated.

**Retinal nerve fiber layer**    Observation of the optic disc remains the key aspect of the clinical examination for glaucoma. However, it has become increasingly evident that examination of the peripapillary retinal nerve fiber layer can provide additional useful information in some circumstances.

The retinal nerve fiber layer can be visualized using achromatic white light, but it is more easily viewed by using a red-free filter. Direct ophthalmoscopy, indirect ophthalmoscopy, and slit-lamp techniques can all be successfully employed to observe the retinal nerve fiber layer. The combination of red-free filter, wide slit beam, and posterior pole lens at the slit lamp affords the best view.

Retinal nerve fiber layer defects can be grouped generally into two broad categories: focal and diffuse. *Focal abnormalities* can consist of slitlike grooves or wedge defects. Slitlike defects can be seen in normal retinal nerve fiber layer anatomy, although they usually do not extend to the disc margin. Early wedge defects are sometimes visible only at a distance from the optic disc margin. *Diffuse nerve fiber loss* is more common in glaucoma than focal loss but also more difficult to observe. Retinal nerve fiber layer photography can often be employed to demonstrate diffuse loss when clinical examination does not.

**Quantitative measurement of the optic nerve head and retinal nerve fiber layer**
The appearance of the optic nerve head has been recognized to be critical in assessing the disease status of glaucoma since the 1850s. However, optic disc assessment can be quite subjective, and inter- and intraobserver variation is greater than desirable given the importance of accurate assessments. Thus, the need for reliable and objective measures of optic disc and associated retinal nerve fiber layer morphology is clear. A number of sophisticated image analysis systems have been developed in recent years to evaluate the optic disc and retinal nerve fiber layer. These instruments give quantitative measurements of various anatomic parameters.

Confocal scanning laser ophthalmoscopy can be utilized to create a three-dimensional image of the optic nerve head. The optical design of instruments using confocal scanning laser technology allows for a series of tomographic "slices," or optical sections, of the structure being imaged. The images acquired by this method are stored as a computer data file and manipulated to reconstruct the three-dimensional structure, display the image, and perform data analysis. Parameters such as cup area, cup volume, rim volume, cup/disc ratio, and peripapillary nerve fiber layer thickness are then calculated.

Techniques such as scanning laser polarimetry and optical coherence tomography (OCT) have been used to acquire images of the retinal nerve fiber layer. The *scanning laser polarimeter* is essentially a scanning laser ophthalmoscope outfitted with a polarization modulator and detector to take advantage of the birefringent properties of the retinal nerve fiber layer arising from the predominantly parallel nature of its microtubule substructure. As light passes through the nerve fiber layer, the polarization state changes. The deeper layers of retinal tissue reflect the light back to the detector where the degree to which the polarization has been changed is recorded. The acquired data can then be stored, displayed, and manipulated by computer programs, as with the unmodified confocal scanning laser ophthalmoscope. The fundamental parameter being measured with this instrumentation is *relative* (not absolute) retinal nerve fiber layer thickness.

*Optical coherence tomography* uses interferometry and low coherence light to obtain a high-resolution cross section of biological structures. The resolution of OCT instrumentation in the eye is approximately 10 µm, and OCT has the potential to yield an absolute measurement of nerve fiber layer thickness. In vivo OCT measurements appear to correlate with histologic measurements of the same tissues.

Quantitative measurement of the optic disc and retinal nerve fiber layer is a promising nascent science. The instrumentation and techniques used to acquire quantitative imaging and analysis of nerve head and nerve fiber layer anatomic parameters are rapidly evolving. The utility of these technologies remains unproven, however, both for single measurements directed at detecting the presence of glaucoma and, especially, for serial measurements necessary to determine clinical progression of glaucoma. The clinician must remember that no system of measurement and observation is currently more useful or proven more reliable than good-quality stereophotographs combined with detailed and careful clinical examination.

Chen YY, Chen PP, Xu L, et al. Correlation of peripapillary nerve fiber layer thickness by scanning laser polarimetry with visual field defects in patients with glaucoma. *J Glaucoma.* 1998;7:312–316.

Wollstein G, Garway-Heath DF, Hitchings RA. Identification of early glaucoma cases with the scanning laser ophthalmoscope. *Ophthalmology.* 1998;105:1557–1563.

***Recording of optic nerve findings***   It is common practice to grade an optic disc by comparing the diameter of the cup to the diameter of the disc. This ratio is usually expressed as a decimal such as 0.2, but such a description poorly conveys the appearance of the nerve head. To avoid confusion the examiner must specify whether the cup is being defined by the change in *color* or in *contour* between the central area of the disc and the surrounding rim. Furthermore, the examiner must specify what is being measured: the horizontal diameter, the vertical diameter, or the longest diameter of the disc. The best description includes the dimensions of the cup specified by both color and contour criteria in both the vertical and horizontal meridians. The rim, which contains the neural elements, should be described in detail: color, width, focal thinning or pallor, and slope. There is a correlation between the rim area and the size of optic disc; i.e., larger optic discs have larger rim areas.

A detailed, annotated diagram of the optic disc topography is preferable to the recording of a simple cup/disc ratio. The diagram must be of adequate size to allow depiction of important topographic landmarks and morphologic features. The diagram with annotation can convey the cup/disc ratio along all dimensions and serves to document the presence or absence of regions of rim thinning, notching, hemorrhage, rim translucency, vessel overpass, and other findings.

The best record of the optic disc is a photograph, preferably stereoscopic and magnified. This record allows the examiner to compare the present status of the patient to baseline status without resorting to memory or grading systems. Moreover, photographs allow better evaluation when a patient has changed doctors. Sometimes subtle optic disc changes become apparent when the clinician compares one set of photographs to a previous set. Careful diagrams of the optic nerve head are useful when photography is not possible or available.

## The Visual Field

The goal of glaucoma management is the preservation of the patient's visual function and quality of life. Visual function is a very complex concept that can be measured in a variety of ways. For many years the standard measurement has been clinical perimetry, which measures differential light sensitivity, or the ability of the subject to distinguish a stimulus light from background illumination. As usually performed in glaucoma examinations, the test uses white light and measures what is conventionally referred to as the *visual field*. The classic description of the visual field given by Harry Moss Traquair (1875–1954), is "an island hill of vision in a sea of darkness."

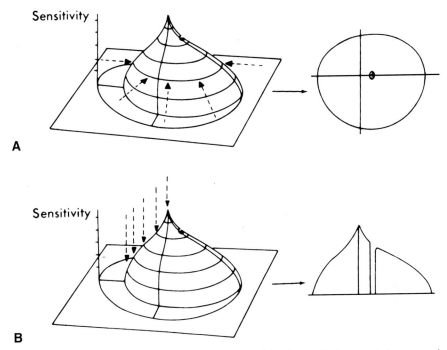

FIG III-16—*A*, Isopter (kinetic) perimetry. Test object of fixed intensity is moved along several meridians toward fixation. Points where the object is first perceived are plotted in a circle. *B,* Static perimetry. Stationary test object is increased in intensity from below threshold until perceived by the patient. Threshold values yield a graphic profile section. (Reproduced with permission from Kolker AE, Hetherington J, eds. *Becker-Shaffer's Diagnosis and Therapy of the Glaucomas.* 5th ed. St Louis: Mosby; 1983. Modified from Aulhorn E, Harms H. In: Leydhecker W. *Glaucoma.* Tutzing Symposium. Basel: S Karger; 1967.)

The island of vision is usually described as a three-dimensional graphic representation of differential light sensitivity at different positions in space (Fig III-16).

*Perimetry* refers to the clinical assessment of the visual field. Perimetry has traditionally served two major purposes in the management of glaucoma:

□ Identification of abnormal fields

□ Quantitative assessment of normal or abnormal fields to guide follow-up care

It has been accepted practice to use the same type of test for both purposes.

A variety of methods have emerged to test visual functions other than differential light sensitivity. The general clinical utility of the newer tests takes time to be established. It is likely that in individual patients, different tests will show abnormalities at different times. Some methods may be better for identification than for follow-up of defects, and vice versa. If, for example, it is true that M cells are selectively damaged early in glaucoma, tests that measure M cell function would perhaps be used for identification of early glaucoma. For the immediate future, however, differential light perimetry with white light will almost certainly continue to be the standard method of identification and follow-up. Other measurements of function that may find a clinical place in glaucoma testing in the future include the following:

□ *Blue/yellow perimetry.* Standard perimeters are available that can project a blue stimulus onto a yellow background. This method seems to be sensitive in the early identification of glaucomatous damage. Several studies suggest that the rate of development of perimetric defects in early glaucoma may be higher with blue on yellow (short wavelength) testing than conventional (achromatic) white on white.

□ *High-pass resolution perimetry.* The stimulus used to test the visual field is a ring-shaped target that varies in size. It is made up of a dark annulus with bright center and dark borders. The average luminance of this target is the same as the background. Thus, the test stimulus is designed to determine spatial resolution thresholds. Test times using high-pass resolution perimetry are shorter than in conventional perimetry.

□ *Frequency doubling perimetry.* This visual field testing paradigm uses a low spatial frequency sinusoidal grating undergoing rapid phase-reversal flicker. Commercially available instruments employ a 0.25 cycles per degree grating phase-reversed at a rapid 25 Hz. When a low spatial frequency grating is presented in this manner, it appears to have twice as many alternating light and dark bars than are actually present, hence the term *frequency doubling.* It is believed that the stimuli employed in this test preferentially activate the M cells and thus may be more sensitive in the detection of early glaucomatous loss.

□ *Contrast sensitivity.* This test measures a subject's ability to detect a pattern of alternating light and dark bands presented at varying frequencies and degrees of contrast.

□ *Flicker sensitivity.* This test measures the ability of the subject to recognize the difference between a flickering light from one that is constantly on. The contrast can be varied.

□ *Visually evoked cortical potentials (VECP,* also *VEP* or *VER)* and *electroretinography (ERG).* Cortical (VECP) or retinal (ERG) electrical responses to a stimulus, such as a reversing pattern of light and dark squares or a flickering light, are recorded. The multifocal ERG may be a useful objective test for assessing retinal ganglion cell function. Although these tests require visual attention, they do not require a subjective response.

Several of these tests are discussed in greater detail in BCSC Section 12, *Retina and Vitreous.*

## Clinical Perimetry

Two major types of perimetry are in general use today:

□ Manual kinetic and static perimetry using a Goldmann-type bowl perimeter
□ Automated static perimetry using a bowl perimeter

Other methods are discussed in standard perimetric texts. In the United States the predominant automated static perimeter is currently the Humphrey Visual Field Analyzer. Most of the clinical examples given are from Humphrey perimeters, and the descriptions apply most directly to that instrument. However, the principles apply to a number of other excellent instruments.

The following are brief definitions of some of the major perimetric terms:

- *Threshold:* The differential light sensitivity at which a stimulus of given size and duration of presentation is seen 50% of the time—in practice, the dimmest spot detected during testing.

- *Suprathreshold:* Above the threshold; generally used to mean brighter than the threshold stimulus. A stimulus may also be made suprathreshold by increasing the size or duration of presentation. This is generally used for screening paradigms.

- *Kinetic testing:* Perimetry in which a target is moved from an area where it is not seen toward an area where it is just seen. This is usually performed manually by a perimetrist who chooses the target, moves it, and records the results.

- *Static testing:* A stationary stimulus is presented at various locations. In theory, the brightness, size, and duration of the stimulus can be varied at each location to determine the threshold. In practice, in a given automated test session, only the brightness is varied. Although static perimetry may be done manually, and is often combined with manual kinetic perimetry, in current practice the term usually refers to automated perimetry.

- *Isopter:* A line on a visual field representation—usually on a two-dimensional sheet of paper—connecting points with the same threshold.

- *Depression:* A decrease in retinal sensitivity.

- *Scotoma:* An area of decreased retinal sensitivity within the visual field surrounded by an area of greater sensitivity.

- *Decibel (dB):* A 0.1 log unit. This is a relative term used in both kinetic and static perimetry that has no absolute value. Its value depends on the maximum illumination of the perimeter. As usually used, it refers to log units of attenuation of the maximum light intensity available in the perimeter being used.

## Patterns of Glaucomatous Nerve Loss

The hallmark defect of glaucoma is the nerve fiber bundle defect that results from damage at the optic nerve head. The pattern of nerve fibers in the retinal area served by the damaged nerve fiber bundle will correspond to the specific defect. The common names for the classic visual field defects are derived from their appearance as plotted on a kinetic visual field chart. In static perimetry, however, the sample points are in a grid pattern, and the representation of visual field defects on a static perimetry chart generally lacks the smooth contours suggested by such terms as *arcuate*.

The following are typical glaucomatous defects that are shown in Figures III-17 through III-21:

- Paracentral scotoma
- Arcuate or Bjerrum scotoma
- Nasal step
- Altitudinal defect
- Temporal wedge

Glaucoma that is far advanced may leave merely a central island of vision (Fig III-22). The superior and inferior poles of the optic nerve appear to be most susceptible to glaucomatous damage. Damage to small scattered bundles throughout the optic nerve head will produce a generalized decrease in sensitivity, which is harder to recognize than focal defects.

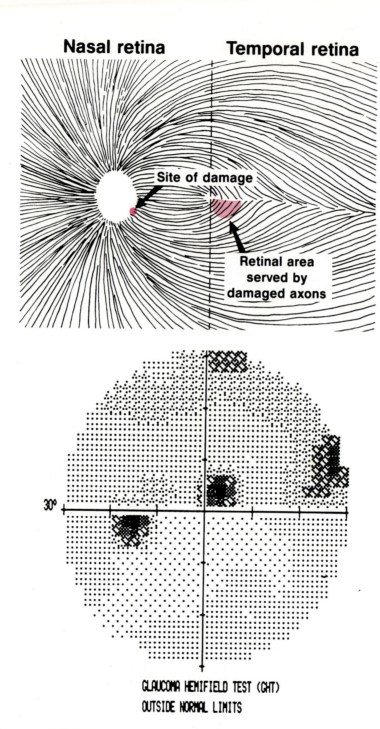

**Nasal retina**　　**Temporal retina**

Site of damage

Retinal area
served by
damaged axons

30°

GLAUCOMA HEMIFIELD TEST (GHT)
OUTSIDE NORMAL LIMITS

FIG III-17—A *paracentral scotoma* is an island of relative or absolute visual loss within 10° of fixation. Loss of nerve fibers from the inferior pole, originating from the inferotemporal retina, resulted in the superonasal scotoma shown. Paracentral scotomata may be single, as in this case, or multiple, and they may occur as isolated findings or may be associated with other early defects (Humphrey 30-2 program).

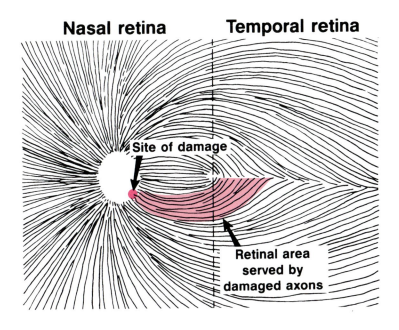

**Nasal retina**  **Temporal retina**

Site of damage

Retinal area
served by
damaged axons

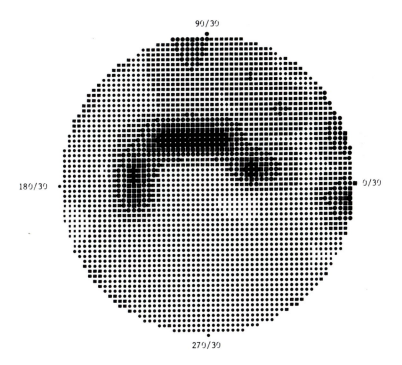

90/30

180/30

0/30

270/30

FIG III-18—An *arcuate scotoma* occurs in the area 10°–20° from fixation. Glaucomatous damage to a nerve fiber bundle that contains axons from both inferonasal and inferotemporal retina resulted in the arcuate defect shown. The scotoma often begins as a single area of relative loss, which then becomes larger, deeper, and multifocal. In its full form an arcuate scotoma arches from the blind spot and ends at the nasal raphe, becoming wider and closer to fixation on the nasal side (Octopus 32 program).

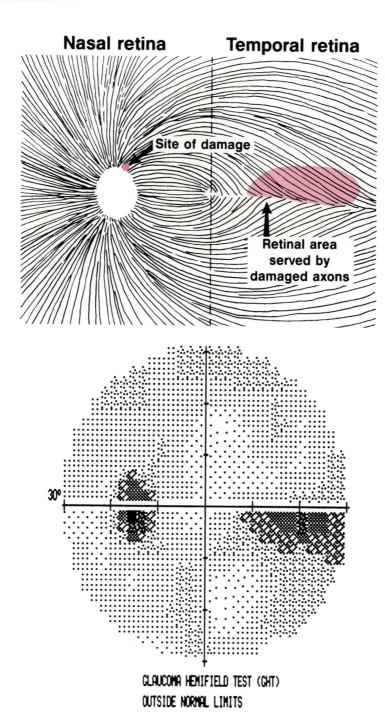

**Nasal retina**　　**Temporal retina**

Site of damage

Retinal area
served by
damaged axons

30°

GLAUCOMA HEMIFIELD TEST (GHT)

OUTSIDE NORMAL LIMITS

FIG III-19—A *nasal step* is a relative depression of one horizontal hemifield compared to the other. Damage to superior nerve fibers serving the superotemporal retina beyond the paracentral area resulted in this nasal step. In kinetic perimetry the nasal step is defined as a discontinuity or depression in one or more nasal isopters near the horizontal raphe (Humphrey 30-2 program).

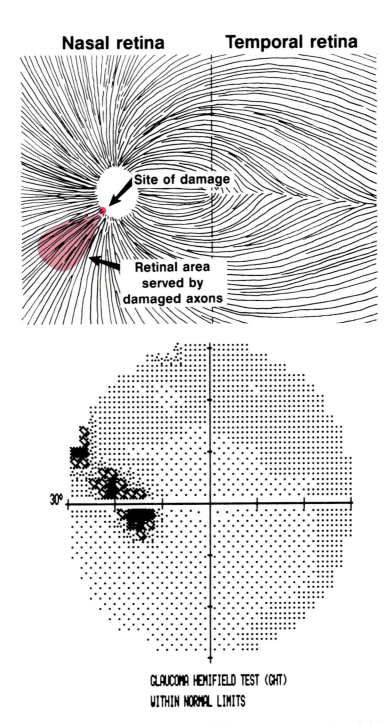

**Nasal retina**　　**Temporal retina**

Site of damage

Retinal area
served by
damaged axons

GLAUCOMA HEMIFIELD TEST (GHT)
WITHIN NORMAL LIMITS

FIG III-20—A *temporal wedge,* also called a *temporal step,* is a wedge-shaped defect that extends temporally from the blind spot or extends from the periphery toward the blind spot. This term is not used to describe defects that extend from the point of fixation or appear to point toward fixation. Damage to the nerve fiber bundle in the inferonasal nerve serving the retina superotemporal to the blind spot produced this temporal wedge. Note that the hemifield test is normal; the test does not include points temporal to the disc (Humphrey 30-2 program).

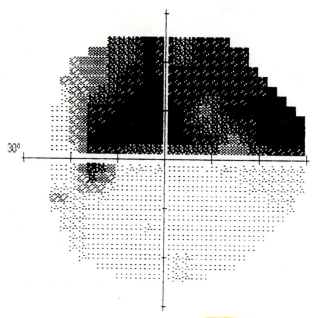

FIG III-21—*Altitudinal defect, left eye.*

| Symb. | dB | asb |
|---|---|---|
| :::  | 51–36 | 0.008–0.25 |
| :::  | 35–31 | 0.31–0.8 |
| ::: | 30–26 | 1–2.5 |
| ::: | 25–21 | 3.1–8 |
| ::: | 20–16 | 10–25 |
| ::: | 15–11 | 31–80 |
| ::: | 10–6 | 100–250 |
| ::: | 5–1 | 315–800 |
| ■ | 0 | 1000 |

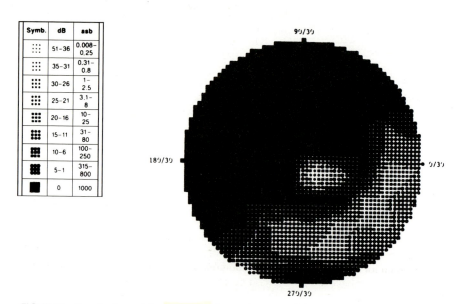

FIG III-22—Examination of the right eye shows dense nasal loss and dense superior loss. Remaining but depressed field is seen inferiorly and superotemporally, and a small island can be seen centrally (Octopus 32 program). (Reproduced with permission from Silverstone DE, Hirsch J. *Automated Visual Field Testing. Techniques of Examination and Interpretation.* East Norwalk, CT: Appleton-Century-Crofts; 1986.)

## Variables in Perimetry

Whether automated or manual, perimetry is subject to many variables, including the human elements involving the patient and the perimetrist.

**Patient**   Humans vary in their attentiveness and response time from moment to moment and from day to day. Longer tests are more likely to produce fatigue and diminish the ability of the patient to maintain peak performance. In addition, retinal sensitivity appears to vary over time. This variability appears to be accentuated in areas of the retina that are abnormal.

**Perimetrist**   The individual performing manual perimetry can administer the test slightly differently each time. Different technicians or physicians also vary from one another. Perimetrist bias is markedly diminished with automated testing. However, the perimetrist can have an effect on test outcome even in automated testing, by monitoring the patient for proper performance and positioning. Most automated instruments can be paused during the test by perimetrist intervention, thereby allowing repositioning or other adjustments to enhance test reliability.

**Other variables**   Other variables of importance include the following:

□ *Fixation:* If the eye is slightly cyclotorted relative to the test bowl, or if the patient's point of fixation is off center, defects may shift locations. Especially in automated static tests (because the test logic does not change), a defect may thus appear and disappear.

□ *Background luminance:* The luminance of the surface onto which the perimetric stimulus is projected affects retinal sensitivity and thus the hill of vision. Clinical perimetry is usually done with a background luminance of 4.0–31.5 apostilbs. Retinal sensitivity is greatest at fixation and falls steadily toward the periphery.

□ *Stimulus luminance:* For a given stimulus size and presentation time, the brighter the stimulus, the more visible.

□ *Size of stimulus:* For a given brightness and duration of presentation, the larger the stimulus, the more likely it is to be perceived. The sizes of standard stimuli are: $0 = 1/16$ mm$^2$, $1 = 1/4$ mm$^2$, $II = 1$ mm$^2$, $III = 4$ mm$^2$, $IV = 16$ mm$^2$, $V = 64$ mm$^2$.

□ *Presentation time:* Fixed on individual automated perimeters. Up to about 0.5 second, temporal summation occurs. In other words, the longer the presentation time, the more visible a given stimulus. Commercially available static perimeters generally employ a stimulus duration of 0.2 seconds or less. Comparison of perimetric thresholds between instruments is difficult since different manufacturers use different stimulus durations and background luminances.

□ *Patient refraction:* Uncorrected refractive errors cause blurring on the retina and decrease the visibility of stimuli. Thus, proper neutralization of refractive errors is essential for accurate perimetry. In addition, presbyopic and many prepresbyopic patients must have a refractive compensation that focuses fixation at the depth of the perimeter bowl.

□ *Pupil size:* Pupil size affects the amount of light entering the eye, and it should be recorded on each field. Testing with pupils smaller than 3 mm in diameter may induce artifacts. Pupil size should be kept constant from test to test.

□ *Wavelength of background and stimulus:* As noted above, color perimetry may yield different results from white-on-white perimetry.

- *Speed of stimulus movement:* Because temporal summation occurs over a time period as long as 0.5 seconds, the area of retina stimulated by a test object is affected by the speed of stimulus movement. If a kinetic target is moved quickly, it may have gone well beyond the location at which it is first seen by the time the patient responds. This period of time between visualization and response is termed the *latency period* or *visual reaction time.*

## Automated Static Perimetry

A computerized perimeter must be able to determine threshold sensitivity at multiple points in the visual field, to perform an adequate test in a reasonable amount of time, and to present results in a comprehensible form. The best instruments currently available are bowl perimeters that project stimuli in programmed locations. The intensity of the stimulus is varied by a system of filters that attenuate the stimulus, usually allowing measurement to approximately 1 dB.

Four general categories of testing strategy are currently in common use:

- *Suprathreshold testing:* A stimulus, usually one expected to be a little brighter than threshold, is presented at various locations and recorded as seen or not seen. Sometimes, if it is not seen, it is presented again, and if not seen a second time, is recorded as not seen. Then the stimulus may be presented at maximum brightness to determine if a defect is relative or absolute. This type of test is designed to screen for moderate to severe defects.

- *Threshold-related strategy:* The threshold is determined at a few points and a presumed hill of vision is extrapolated from these points. Then a stimulus 6 dB brighter is presented, and the results are recorded as either seen or not seen. This type of test will detect moderate to severe defects, but it may miss mild defects (Fig III-23).

- *Threshold:* Threshold testing is the current standard for automated perimetry in glaucoma management. Threshold may be determined by a variety of bracketing and statistical strategies (Fig III-24). Usually, several points are tested twice to determine a patient's variability, and occasional tests are done to monitor fixation and to assess the frequency of a given individual's false-positive and false-negative responses.

- *SITA:* Full threshold testing algorithms suffer from patient fatigue, high variability, and generally poor patient acceptance. Although shorter threshold testing algorithms such as FASTPAC have been developed, the variability of the results of these shorter tests remains a concern that tempers confidence in their results. In an attempt to achieve shorter threshold testing with good accuracy and reproducibility, the Swedish Interactive Thresholding Algorithm (SITA) was developed. This testing algorithm takes advantage of current knowledge regarding visual field sensitivity and mathematical modeling and estimation of threshold values. Threshold values and measurement errors are continuously estimated during the test using maximum posterior probability calculations developed from visual field models. During testing, the stair-step procedures used to determine threshold sensitivity may be interrupted when the measurement error appears to have reached a predetermined level, thus decreasing the number of stimuli presented and reducing the test duration. Test time is also shortened by elimination of the catch trials for false-positive responses and use of a more effective timing algorithm for presentation of the different stimuli.

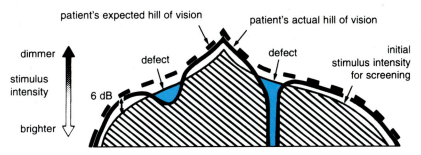

FIG III-23—Threshold-related screening strategy records tested points as seen or not seen. Screening is done at an intensity 6 dB brighter than the expected threshold, and points missed twice at that level are recorded as defects. (Reproduced with permission from *The Field Analyzer Primer.* San Leandro, CA: Allergan Humphrey; 1989.)

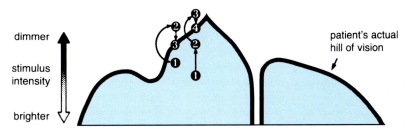

FIG III-24—Full-threshold strategy determines retinal sensitivity at each tested point by altering the stimulus intensity in 4-dB steps until the threshold is crossed. It then recrosses the threshold, moving in 2-dB steps, in order to check and refine the accuracy of the measurement. (Reproduced with permission from *The Field Analyzer Primer.* San Leandro, CA: Allergan Humphrey; 1989.)

Comparisons between SITA testing algorithms and older thresholding algorithms have suggested that the SITA Standard yields visual field results comparable to full threshold testing, while the SITA Fast algorithm is comparable to FASTPAC. Both SITA strategies yield marginally higher values for differential light sensitivity compared with other algorithms, but visual field defects are statistically deeper and better defined, most likely because the decrease in patient fatigue reduces variability both within the test and between tests. Average test time with SITA Standard is approximately 50% the full thresholding strategy time, and SITA Fast results in an additional reduction of approximately 30% compared with SITA Standard. The significantly reduced test time with SITA Standard appears to be achieved without sacrifice of accuracy or increase in variability or noise levels within the test. In addition, with the normative database, the probability plots and their probability limits for normality appear to be tighter with SITA than with standard threshold testing algorithms. This quality may allow for earlier separation of normals from abnormals at an earlier stage and may allow for better detection for change over time.

Of the many tests available, only a few are generally used in glaucoma management. The clinician's degree of suspicion and the individual's known status as glaucoma suspect, nonsuspect, or patient guide the choice of instrument.

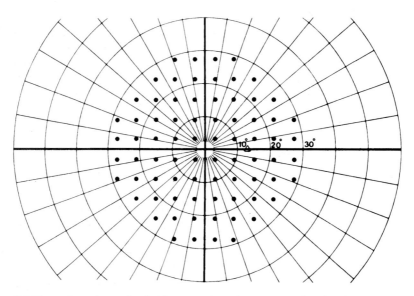

FIG III-25—Central 30-2 threshold test pattern, right eye. (Reproduced with permission from *The Field Analyzer Primer.* San Leandro, CA: Allergan Humphrey; 1989.)

***Screening tests*** These tests may or may not be threshold related, and they cover varying areas of the visual field. Suprathreshold tests are not recommended for glaucoma suspects, since they do not provide a good reference for future comparison, but they are appropriate for screening people not suspected of having glaucoma. On a full-field screening test, such as the Octopus 07 or Humphrey full-field 120-point test, a field should be considered abnormal if more than 10 points are missed or if 2 or more adjacent points are missed. A threshold field should be performed on such patients unless a cause other than glaucoma is apparent on examination.

***Threshold tests*** The most common programs for glaucoma testing are the central 24° and 30° programs, such as the Octopus 32 and G1 and the Humphrey 24-2 and 30-2 (Fig III-25). These programs test the central field using a 6° grid. They test points 3° above and 3° below the horizontal midline and facilitate diagnosis of defects that respect this line.

Although a 30°–60° program is available on most static threshold perimeters, it is rarely performed. The abandonment of peripheral testing that has accompanied the shift from manual to automated perimetry is the subject of ongoing discussion, but no trend to move beyond the central program has emerged after more than two decades of static threshold perimetry. In part, at least, this pattern of use is related to a subtle change in the role of the visual field examination. The automated static threshold field determines retinal sensitivity at a preset series of points. If a defect is found, it is not plotted precisely as it would be with manual perimetry. Ideally, an abnormal field is repeated, and the result is a precise map of sensitivity at selected locations. In practice, this method appears to be superior to kinetic testing for following a patient over time.

## Interpretation of a Single Field

**Quality**   The first aspect of the field to be evaluated is its quality. The percentage of fixation losses, the false positives and false negatives, and the fluctuations of doubly determined points are assessed. Damaged areas of the field demonstrate more variability than normal areas. Glaucomatous damage may cause an increase in false-negative responses unrelated to patient reliability. In general, the average fluctuation between two determinations should be less than 2 dB in a normal field, less than 3 dB in a field with early damage, and less than 4 dB in a field with moderate damage. Patient reliability can be evaluated by looking at the least damaged areas in a badly damaged visual field.

**Normality or abnormality**   Next to be assessed is the normality or abnormality. When tested under photopic conditions, the normal visual field demonstrates the greatest sensitivity centrally, with sensitivity falling steadily toward the periphery. A cluster of two or more points depressed ≥5 dB compared with surrounding points is suspicious. A single point depressed >10 dB is very unusual but is of less value on a single visual field than a cluster, because cluster points confirm one another. Corresponding points above and below the horizontal midline should not vary markedly; normally the superior field is depressed 1–2 dB compared with the inferior field.

To aid the clinician in interpreting the numerical data generated by threshold tests, field indices have been developed by perimeter manufacturers. In addition to the mean difference from normal and the test-retest variability, other measures of the irregularity of the visual field include Humphrey pattern standard deviation and Octopus loss variance indices. These indices highlight localized depressions in the field. When corrected for short-term fluctuation, the indices are termed *corrected pattern standard deviation* and *corrected loss variance*.

These corrected indices help to distinguish between generalized field depression and localized loss. An abnormal pattern deviation has greater diagnostic specificity than a generalized loss of sensitivity. An abnormally high pattern standard deviation indicates that some points of the visual field are depressed relative to other points in the field after correction for the patient's moment-to-moment variability. Such a finding is suggestive of focal damage such as that occurring with glaucoma (and many other conditions). Although a normal pattern standard deviation in an eye with an abnormal visual field indicates a generalized depression of the hill of vision such as that occurring with media opacity, such generalized loss may also occur with diffuse glaucomatous damage.

The Humphrey STATPAC 2 program performs an additional calculation on a single field to determine the likelihood that a field shows glaucomatous damage. This test is designed only for glaucoma and involves comparison of corresponding points above and below the horizontal midline (Fig III-26). This hemifield analysis is at least as accurate as other methods for the classification of single visual fields.

**Artifacts**   Identification of artifacts is the next step in evaluating the visual field. The following are common artifacts seen on automated perimetry:

□ *Lens rim:* If the patient's corrective lens is decentered or set too far from the eye, the lens rim may project into the central 30° (Fig III-27).

□ *Incorrect corrective lens:* If an incorrect corrective lens is used, the resulting field will be generally depressed. In practice, such an error is rarely noted, but it probably accounts for the occasional inexplicably depressed field that improves on follow-up testing.

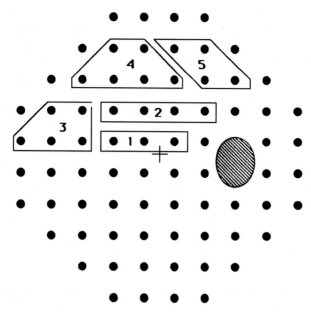

FIG III-26—Superior field zones used in the glaucoma hemifield test. (Reproduced with permission from *The STATPAC User's Guide.* San Leandro, CA: Allergan Humphrey; 1989.)

□ *Cloverleaf field:* If a patient stops paying attention and ceases to respond partway through a visual field, a distinctive field pattern may develop, depending on the test logic of a given perimeter. Figure III-28 shows a cloverleaf field, the result of the test logic of the Humphrey 30-2 perimeter, which begins testing with the points circled and works outward.

□ *High false-positive rate:* When a patient responds at a time when no test stimulus is being presented, a false-positive response is recorded. False-positive rates greater than 33% suggest unreliability of the test. A high false-positive response rate can in extreme cases result in a field with impossibly high threshold values (Fig III-29). A high false-positive and a high fixation-loss rate will also occur if the instrument records fixation losses by presenting stimuli in the blind spot. Careful instruction of the patient may sometimes resolve this artifact.

□ *High false-negative rate:* When a patient fails to respond to a stimulus presented in a location where a dimmer stimulus was previously seen, a false-negative response is recorded. False-negative rates greater than 33% suggest unreliability of the test. A high false-negative rate should alert the clinician to the likelihood that the patient's actual visual field might not be as depressed as suggested by the test result. However, it should also be noted that patients with significant visual field loss including scotomata with steep edges can demonstrate high false-negative rates that do not indicate unreliability. This effect appears to arise from presentation of stimuli at the edges of deep scotomata where short-term fluctuation of threshold can be quite variable.

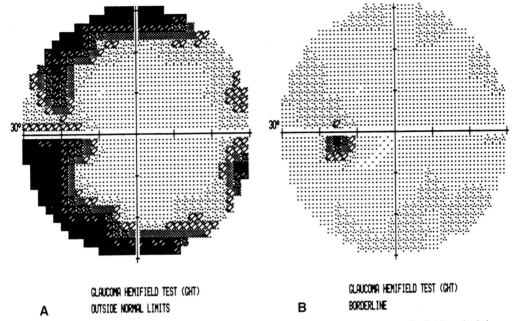

FIG III-27—Lens rim artifact. The two visual fields shown were obtained 9 days apart. The field on the left, A, shows a typical lens rim artifact, whereas the corrective lens was positioned appropriately for the field on the right, B (Humphrey 30-2 program).

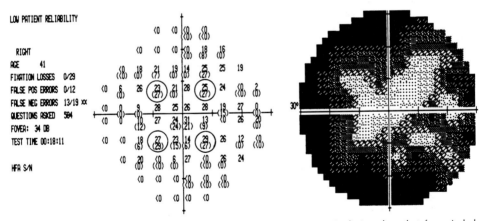

FIG III-28—Cloverleaf field. The Humphrey visual field perimeter test is designed so that four circled points are checked initially and the testing in each quadrant proceeds outward from these points. If the patient ceases to respond after only a few points have been tested, the result is some variation of the cloverleaf field shown at right (Humphrey 30-2 program).

DATE   10-02-86

## DATE   10-02-86

LOW PATIENT RELIABILITY

LEFT
AGE        52
FIXATION LOSSES    24/33 xx
FALSE POS ERRORS   9/23 xx
FALSE NEG ERRORS   8/21 xx
QUESTIONS ASKED    689
FOVEA:  33 DB ::
TEST TIME 00:22:31

HFA S/N

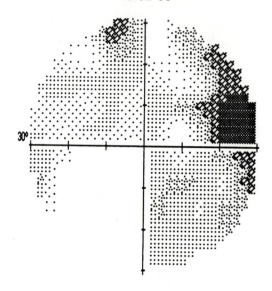

GLAUCOMA HEMIFIELD TEST (GHT)
ABNORMALLY HIGH SENSITIVITY

## DATE   10-23-86

LEFT
AGE        52
FIXATION LOSSES    1/27
FALSE POS ERRORS   0/18
FALSE NEG ERRORS   0/13
QUESTIONS ASKED    516
FOVEA:  30 DB ■
TEST TIME 00:15:03

HFA S/N

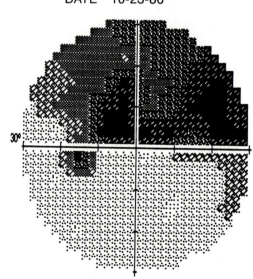

GLAUCOMA HEMIFIELD TEST (GHT)
OUTSIDE NORMAL LIMITS

FIG III-29—High false-positive rate. The top visual field contains characteristic "white sco-tomata," which represent areas of impossibly high retinal sensitivity. Upon return visit 3 weeks later, the patient was carefully instructed to respond only when she saw the light, resulting in the bottom visual field, which shows good reliability and demonstrates the patient's dense superior visual field loss (Humphrey 30-2 program).

## Interpretation of a Series of Fields

Interpretation of serial visual fields should meet two goals:

□ Separating real change from ordinary variation

□ Using the information from the field testing to determine the likelihood that a change is related to glaucomatous progression

A number of methods can be employed in the analysis of a series of visual fields for glaucomatous change. Point-by-point analysis by hand, in the absence of a statistical program package, is extremely cumbersome. The mountain of data present in a series of visual fields cannot be effectively analyzed by hand. Fortunately, statistical programs are available from the major instrument manufacturers (for example, the Humphrey STATPAC 2 or Octopus Delta programs), and these are valuable aids in point-by-point series analysis. The application of each of these packages is described clearly in the owner's manual that comes with the program.

Calculation and comparison of visual field indices is another method that can be useful in visual field series analysis. Examination of visual field indices can reveal global trends that may be missed using point-by-point analysis. Raw perimetric data can also be transferred to independent software programs for change analysis. Even when computed statistical methods are employed, separation of true pathologic progression from normal test-to-test variability remains a difficult challenge. Moreover, the examiner interpreting a series of visual fields must keep in mind that test variability is increased as part of the pathophysiology of glaucoma.

Whatever method the clinician uses, the fundamental requirement for adequate interpretation over time is a good *baseline* visual field. Often the patient experiences a learning effect, and the second visual field may show substantial improvement over the first (Fig III-30). At least two visual fields should be obtained as early in a patient's course as possible. If they are quite different, a third test should be performed. Subsequent visual fields should be compared to these baseline fields. Any follow-up visual field that appears to be quite different should be repeated for confirmation of the suspected change from baseline.

***Progression*** No hard-and-fast rules define what determines visual field progression, but the following are reasonable guidelines:

□ Deepening of an existing scotoma is suggested by the reproducible depression of a point in an existing scotoma by ≥7 dB

□ Enlargement of an existing scotoma is suggested by the reproducible depression of a point adjacent to an existing scotoma by ≥9 dB

□ Development of a new scotoma is suggested by the reproducible depression of a previously normal point in the visual field by ≥11 dB, or of two adjacent previously normal points by ≥5 dB

Cases such as that shown in Figure III-31 are easy to recognize. A general decrease in sensitivity may be secondary to glaucoma or may be related to media opacity, and clinical correlation is required, which is often difficult. Two causes of general decline in sensitivity that may confuse interpretation are variable miosis (often related to use of eyedrops) and cataract (Fig III-32). To help avoid this problem, the pupil size should remain constant from field to field if at all possible.

***Correlation with optic disc*** It is important to correlate changes in the visual field with the optic disc. If such correlation is lacking, other causes of visual loss should

DATE 09-14-90

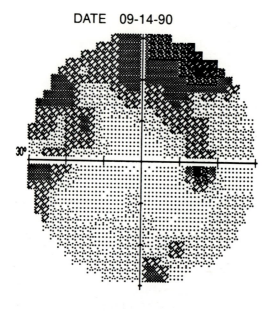

GLAUCOMA HEMIFIELD TEST (GHT)
OUTSIDE NORMAL LIMITS

DATE 10-05-90

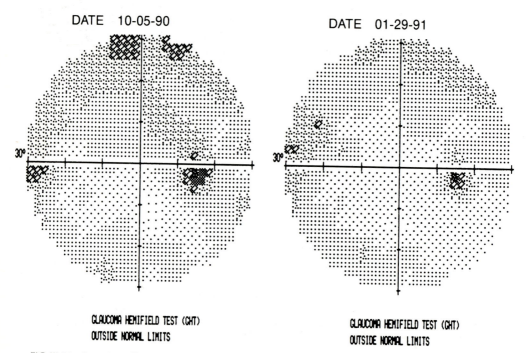

GLAUCOMA HEMIFIELD TEST (GHT)
OUTSIDE NORMAL LIMITS

DATE 01-29-91

GLAUCOMA HEMIFIELD TEST (GHT)
OUTSIDE NORMAL LIMITS

FIG III-30—Learning effect. These three visual fields were obtained within the first 3½ months of diagnosis in a patient with very early, clinically stable, glaucoma. They illustrate the learning effect between the first and second visual field. The third field is similar to the second field, and the second and third visual fields provided a baseline for subsequent follow-up of the patient (Humphrey 30-2 program).

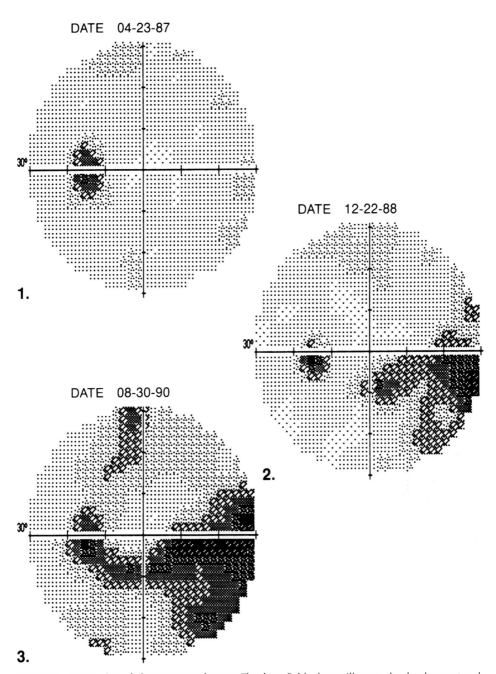

DATE 04-23-87

1.

DATE 12-22-88

2.

DATE 08-30-90

3.

FIG III-31—Progression of glaucomatous damage. The three fields shown illustrate the development and advancement of a visual field defect. Between the first and second visual fields, the patient developed a significant inferior nasal step. The third visual field illustrates the extension of this defect to the blind spot, as well as the development of superior visual field loss (Humphrey 30-2 program).

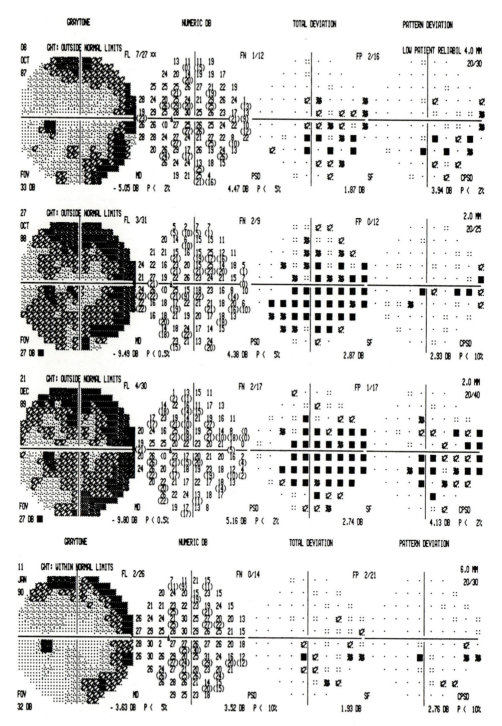

FIG III-32—Pupil size. The first field in this series was obtained before the patient began pilocarpine therapy. The second and third fields were obtained with a miotic pupil. Before the fourth field was obtained, the patient's pupil was dilated (Humphrey 30-2 program).

be considered, such as ischemic optic neuropathy, demyelinating or other neuro-logic disease, pituitary tumor, and so on. This consideration is especially important in the following situations:

□ The patient's optic disc seems less cupped than would be expected for the degree of field loss

□ The pallor of the disc is more impressive than the cupping

□ The progression of the visual field loss seems excessive

□ The pattern of visual field loss is uncharacteristic for glaucoma, e.g., respecting the vertical midline

Anderson DR, Patella VM. *Automated Static Perimetry.* 2nd ed. St Louis: Mosby; 1992.

Drake MV. A primer on automated perimetry. In: *Focal Points: Clinical Modules for Ophthalmologists.* San Francisco: American Academy of Ophthalmology; 1993: vol 11, no 8.

Drance SM, Anderson DR, eds. *Automatic Perimetry in Glaucoma: A Practical Guide.* Orlando, Fla: Grune & Stratton; 1985.

Harrington DO, Drake MV. *The Visual Fields: A Textbook and Atlas of Clinical Perimetry.* 6th ed. St Louis: Mosby; 1989.

Lieberman MF. Glaucoma and automated perimetry. *In: Focal Points: Clinical Modules for Ophthalmologists.* San Francisco: American Academy of Ophthalmology; 1993: vol 11, no 9.

Walsh TJ, ed. *Visual Fields: Examination and Interpretation.* 2nd ed. Ophthalmology Monograph 3. San Francisco: American Academy of Ophthalmology; 1996.

## Manual Perimetry

The two goals of perimetry—to identify abnormalities and to define and record visual function for comparison over time—are most commonly pursued in manual perimetry using *the Armaly-Drance screening technique.* This screening technique for the detection of early glaucomatous visual field loss was originally developed for the Goldmann perimeter but has been adapted for a number of instruments. It combines a kinetic examination of the peripheral isopters with a suprathreshold static examination of the central field (Fig III-33).

With this technique the kinetic perimeter—usually the Goldmann I–2e—is used to determine the stimulus that is just suprathreshold for the central 25°. The central isopter is then plotted kinetically with this stimulus to detect nasal, temporal, or vertical steps, with special attention to the 15° straddling the horizontal and vertical meridians. The blind spot is mapped with the same stimulus moving from the center of the blind spot outward in eight directions. The same stimulus is then used in static presentations to search for paracentral and arcuate defects. A more intense stimulus, often the equivalent of a Goldmann I–4e, is used to search for both nasal step and temporal sector defects to prepare a kinetic plot of the peripheral isopter.

A different perimetric technique must be used for quantifying defects and for following patients with established glaucomatous damage. This form of perimetry quantifies visual field defects by size, shape, and depth and determines whether the disease is progressing or not. If the examiner is using a kinetic technique, targets of different size and brightness must be employed. The technique of quantifying defects with kinetic perimetry is well described in standard texts. An example of a quantified defect is shown in Figure III-34.

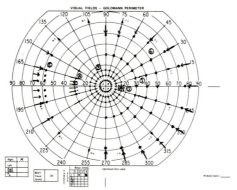

FIG III-33—Armaly-Drance screening technique on Goldmann perimeter.

Progression of glaucomatous field loss generally occurs in areas damaged previously. Scotomata become larger and deeper, and new scotomata appear in the same hemifield. Arcuate scotomata extend to the peripheral boundaries on the nasal side and break through to the periphery. The ophthalmologist who quantifies defects with precision can use this pattern of progression to determine a patient's ongoing stability or progression.

Since high-quality manual threshold perimetry requires a well-trained and conscientious perimetrist, and even the best perimetrist varies from day to day, automated field testing has become increasingly widespread. Computerized static perimetry has shown itself to be at least as good as the best-quality manual perimetry in the detection and quantification of glaucomatous defects. However, manual perimetry remains helpful in documenting defects outside the central 30° and in monitoring endstage visual field loss.

Anderson DR. *Perimetry With and Without Automation.* 2nd ed. St Louis: Mosby; 1987.

## Other Tests

Several other tests may be helpful in selected patients. Many of these tests are described elsewhere in the BCSC series, and the reader is advised to consult the *Master Index* for the following:

- Fluorescein angiography
- Corneal pachymetry
- Measurement of episcleral venous pressure
- Ophthalmodynamometry
- Carotid noninvasive vascular studies
- Ocular blood-flow measurements
- Ultrasonography

Although it is not currently widely available, ultrasound biomicroscopy (UBM) provides valuable information about several types of glaucoma. The test employs shorter wavelength sound waves than does conventional ocular ultrasound, limiting the penetration but increasing the resolution tenfold. The test allows detailed examination of the anterior segment, the posterior chamber, and the ciliary body (Fig III-35).

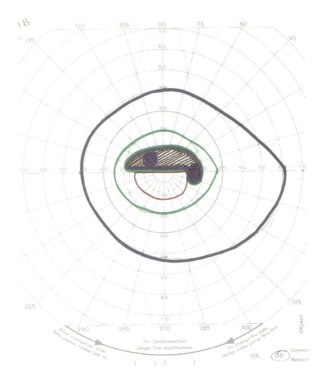

FIG III-34—Split fixation (Goldmann perimeter).

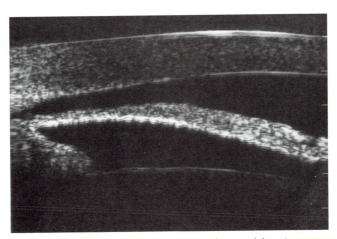

FIG III-35—**Pupillary block** as shown by **ultrasound biomicroscopy.** Note the elevation above the lens of the peripheral iris on the left compared with the central iris on the right. (Photograph courtesy of Charles J. Pavlin, MD.)

# CHAPTER IV

# Open-Angle Glaucoma

## Primary Open-Angle Glaucoma

Primary open-angle glaucoma (POAG) is a chronic, slowly progressive optic neuropathy characterized by atrophy and cupping of the optic nerve head and associated with characteristic patterns of visual field loss. IOP is an important risk factor for primary open-angle glaucoma, and other factors such as race, age, and family history also contribute to the risk of development of this disease. In addition, reduced blood supply to the optic nerve, abnormalities of axonal or ganglion cell metabolism, and disorders of the extracellular matrix of the lamina cribrosa may be contributory factors. Unfortunately, the puzzle of the interplay of multifactorial causes of POAG remains unsolved.

### Clinical Features

Primary open-angle glaucoma is usually insidious in onset, slowly progressive, and painless. While usually bilateral, it can be quite asymmetric. Because central visual acuity is relatively unaffected until late in the disease, visual loss generally progresses without symptoms. Primary open-angle glaucoma is diagnosed by assessing a combination of findings including IOP levels, optic disc appearance, and visual field loss, as illustrated in chapter III.

***Intraocular Pressure*** Large, population-based epidemiologic studies have revealed a mean IOP of approximately 16 mm Hg, with a standard deviation of approximately 3 mm Hg. The range of normal IOP has been defined as 2 standard deviations above and below the mean IOP, or approximately 10–22 mm Hg.

Although IOP greater than 22 mm Hg has often been defined as "abnormal," this definition has a number of shortcomings. First, it is now known that IOP in a general population is not represented by a gaussian distribution but is skewed toward higher pressures (see Figure II-3). IOPs of 22 mm Hg and above would thus not necessarily represent abnormality from a statistical standpoint. More important, IOP distribution curves in glaucomatous and nonglaucomatous eyes show a great deal of overlap. An IOP cutoff value of 21 or 22 mm Hg thus has no real clinical significance. Several studies have indicated that as many as 30%–50% of individuals in the general population who have glaucomatous optic neuropathy and/or visual field loss have initial screening IOPs below 22 mm Hg. Furthermore, because of diurnal fluctuation, elevations of IOP may occur only intermittently in some glaucomatous eyes, with as many as one third of the measurements being normal. The IOP in an untreated glaucoma patient may vary rapidly, by 15 mm Hg or more, over a 24-hour period.

***Optic disc appearance and visual field loss*** Although elevated IOP is still considered a key risk factor for glaucoma, it is no longer considered essential to its diag-

Table IV-1

Controlled Clinical Trials with Published Results

| NAME/DATE OF PUBLISHED RESULTS | STUDY DESIGN | RECRUITMENT (NO. OF PATIENTS) | FOLLOW-UP DURATION (YEARS) | FINDING |
|---|---|---|---|---|
| Scottish Glaucoma Trial/1989 | Newly diagnosed POAG: medicine vs trabeculectomy | 99 | 3–5 | Trabeculectomy lowered IOP more than medicine; medicine group lost more visual function than trabeculectomy group. |
| Moorfields Primary Treatment Trial/1994 | Newly diagnosed POAG: medicine vs laser trabeculoplasty vs trabeculectomy | 168 | 5+ | Trabeculectomy lowered IOP the most; laser trabeculoplasty and medicine groups lost more visual function than trabeculectomy group. |
| Glaucoma Laser Trial (GLT)/1990 | Newly diagnosed POAG: medicine vs laser trabeculoplasty | 271 | 2.5–5.5 | Initial laser trabeculoplasty is at least as effective as initial treatment with topical timolol maleate to reduce IOP and preserve vision. |
| Glaucoma Laser Trial Follow-up Study/1995 | Participants in the GLT | 203 | 6–9 | Initial laser trabeculoplasty is at least as effective as initial treatment with topical timolol maleate to reduce IOP and preserve vision. |
| Fluorouracil Filtering Surgery Study/1989, 1996 | Patients at high risk for surgical failure: results of trabeculectomy with or without 5-fluorouracil | 213 | 5+ | Substantial improvements in IOP reduction with adjunctive 5-fluorouracil. |
| Normal-Tension Glaucoma Study/1998 | POAG in eyes with normal IOP: rate of progression, effect of IOP reduction on progression rate | 200 | 5+ | Lowering IOP retards the progression rate of visual field loss compared with untreated eyes. |
| Advanced Glaucoma Intervention Study/1998 | POAG after medical treatment failure with no previous surgery: laser trabeculoplasty vs trabeculectomy | 591 (789 eyes) | 4–7 | Surgical outcome varies by race; African American patients do better with trabeculoplasty as first surgery, while in the longer term (4+ years) white patients do better with trabeculectomy. |

Modified from Preferred Practice Patterns Committee, Glaucoma Panel. *Primary Open-Angle Glaucoma.* San Francisco: American Academy of Ophthalmology; 2000.

nosis. Optic nerve head appearance and visual field defects have assumed predominant roles in the diagnosis of primary open-angle glaucoma, although treatment at this time remains aimed at lowering the IOP. Tables IV-1 and IV-2 summarize current clinical trials to evaluate control of IOP and POAG.

Careful periodic evaluation of the optic disc and visual field is vital in follow-up of glaucoma patients. Stereophotographic documentation or computerized imag-

TABLE IV-2

CONTROLLED CLINICAL TRIALS IN PROGRESS

| NAME/DATE | STUDY DESIGN | RECRUITMENT GOALS (NO. OF PATIENTS) | PROJECTED FOLLOW-UP (YEARS) |
|---|---|---|---|
| Ocular Hypertension Treatment Study/1999 | Ocular hypertensive patients: medicine vs no treatment | 1500 | 5+ |
| Advanced Glaucoma Intervention Study/1994 | POAG after medical treatment failure with no previous surgery: laser trabeculoplasty vs trabeculectomy | 591 (789 eyes) | 10 |
| Early Manifest Glaucoma Trial/1999 | Newly diagnosed POAG: medicine and laser trabeculoplasty vs no treatment | 300 | 4+ |
| Collaborative Initial Glaucoma Treatment Study/1999 | Newly diagnosed POAG: medicine vs trabeculectomy | 600 | 5+ |

Modified from Preferred Practice Patterns Committee, Glaucoma Panel. *Primary Open-Angle Glaucoma.* San Francisco: American Academy of Ophthalmology; 2000.

ing of the disc enhances the clinician's ability to detect subtle changes on follow-up. Pertinent clinical signs of glaucoma in the optic disc include the following:

- ☐ Asymmetry of the neuroretinal rim area or cupping
- ☐ Focal thinning or notching of the neuroretinal rim
- ☐ Optic disc hemorrhage
- ☐ Especially, any acquired change in the disc rim appearance or the surrounding retinal nerve fiber layer

An attempt should be made to correlate changes in the optic disc with defects in the visual field.

Gonioscopy should be performed in all patients evaluated for glaucoma and repeated periodically in open-angle glaucoma patients to detect possible progressive angle closure caused by miotic therapy or age-related lens changes, especially in hyperopic patients. Repeat gonioscopy is also indicated when the chamber becomes shallow, when strong miotics are prescribed, after laser trabeculoplasty or iridectomy, and when IOP rises.

***Risk factors for POAG Other Than IOP*** *Race* is an important risk factor for POAG. The prevalence of POAG is four to five times greater in African Americans than in others, and a similar prevalence is present in the black inhabitants of Barbados (Table IV-3). Blindness from glaucoma is four to eight times more common in African Americans than in white residents of the United States.

*Age* is another important risk factor for the presence of POAG. The Baltimore Eye Survey found that the prevalence of glaucoma increases dramatically with age, particularly among African Americans, exceeding 11% in those 80 years of age or older.

*Family history* is also a risk factor for glaucoma. The Baltimore Eye Survey found that the relative risk of having POAG is increased approximately 3.7-fold for individuals having a sibling with POAG.

TABLE IV-3

PREVALENCE OF DEFINITE
PRIMARY OPEN-ANGLE GLAUCOMA BY AGE AND RACE

| AGE (YEARS) | NO. SCREENED | NO. OF CASES | OBSERVED RATE/ 100 (95% CI)* | ADJUSTED RATE/ 100 (95% CI) |
|---|---|---|---|---|
| **White Americans** | | | | |
| 40–49 | 543 | 1 | 0.18 (0.02–1.03) | 0.92 (0–2.72) |
| 50–59 | 618 | 2 | 0.32 (0.03–1.17) | 0.41 (0–0.98) |
| 60–69 | 915 | 7 | 0.77 (0.31–1.57) | 0.88 (0.14–1.62) |
| 70–79 | 631 | 18 | 2.85 (1.70–4.50) | 2.89 (1.44–4.34) |
| ≥80 | 206 | 4 | 1.94 (0.49–4.95) | 2.16 (0.05–4.26) |
| Total | 2913 | 32 | 1.10 (0.75–1.55) | 1.29 (0.80–1.78) |
| **African Americans** | | | | |
| 40–49 | 632 | 6 | 0.95 (0.35–2.07) | 1.23 (0.23–2.24) |
| 50–59 | 699 | 25 | 3.58 (2.32–5.26) | 4.05 (2.47–5.63) |
| 60–69 | 614 | 31 | 5.05 (3.42–7.17) | 5.51 (3.57–7.46) |
| 70–79 | 349 | 27 | 7.74 (4.94–10.54) | 9.15 (5.83–12.48) |
| ≥80 | 101 | 11 | 10.89 (4.81–16.97) | 11.26 (4.52–18.00) |
| Total | 2395 | 100 | 4.18 (3.38–4.98) | 4.74 (3.81–5.67) |

Modified from Tielsch JM, Sommer A, Katz J, et al. Racial variations in the prevalence of primary open-angle glaucoma. The Baltimore Eye Survey. *JAMA.* 1991;266:369–374.

*CI = confidence interval.

## Associated Disorders

Some of the conditions described below are discussed in greater detail elsewhere in the BCSC series. See also Section 1, *Update on General Medicine* (diabetes and cardiovascular disease), and Section 12, *Retina and Vitreous* (diabetes and retinal vein occlusion).

**Myopia**   An association between POAG and myopia has been reported. It is possible that myopic individuals may be at increased risk for the development of glaucoma. Another possible explanation is that the association between myopia and primary open-angle glaucoma is influenced by selection bias, since persons who have refractive errors are more likely to seek eye care and thus have a higher probability than emmetropic individuals of having glaucoma detected early.

The concurrence of POAG and myopia may complicate both diagnosis and management. Disc evaluation is particularly complicated in the presence of myopic fundus changes, such as tilting of the disc and posterior staphylomas, that may make an assessment of cupping difficult. Myopia-related retinal changes can cause visual field abnormalities apart from any glaucomatous process. High refractive error may also make it difficult to perform accurate perimetric measurement and to interpret visual field abnormalities. In addition, the magnification of the disc associated with the myopic refractive error interferes with optic disc evaluation.

***Diabetes mellitus***   Studies have reported a higher prevalence of both elevated mean IOP and of primary open-angle glaucoma among persons with diabetes compared with those without diabetes. In addition, glaucoma patients have been reported to have a higher prevalence of abnormal glucose metabolism than the general population. Some authorities believe that the small-vessel involvement in diabetes makes the optic disc more susceptible to pressure-related damage.

***Cardiovascular disease***   Positive associations between blood pressure and IOP and between blood pressure and POAG have been reported. The hypothesis that systemic hypertension, with its possible microcirculatory effects on the optic disc, may increase susceptibility to glaucoma is biologically plausible. However, evidence that cardiovascular disease is a risk factor for glaucoma is weak. The possible role of arteriosclerotic and ischemic vascular disease is also unclear, but these factors may be important in the development of some cases of glaucoma, particularly those with IOP in the normal range. Evidence is accumulating that suggests vascular autoregulatory abnormalities in individuals with glaucoma, and ongoing research into the pathophysiology of glaucoma may expand on these findings in the future.

***Retinal vein occlusion***   Patients with central retinal vein occlusion (CRVO) may present with elevated IOP or glaucoma. This relationship may be obscured by the temporary hypotony that often follows the vein occlusion. In susceptible individuals, eyes with elevated IOP are at risk of developing CRVO. Thus, elevated IOP in the fellow eye of an eye affected with retinal vein occlusion must be kept as low as reasonably possible.

Schwartz B. Optic disc evaluation in glaucoma. In: *Focal Points: Clinical Modules for Ophthalmologists.* San Francisco: American Academy of Ophthalmology; 1990: vol 8, no 12.

## The Glaucoma Suspect

A glaucoma suspect is defined as an adult who has one of the following findings in at least one eye:

☐ An optic nerve or nerve fiber layer suggestive of glaucoma (enlarged cup/disc ratio, asymmetric cup/disc ratio, notching or narrowing of the neural rim, a disc hemorrhage, or diffuse or local abnormality in the nerve fiber layer)

☐ A suspicious visual field abnormality

☐ An elevated IOP consistently greater than 22 mm Hg

Usually, if two or more of these findings are present, the diagnosis of primary open-angle glaucoma is supported, especially in the presence of other risk factors such as advanced age (>50), family history of glaucoma, and African American descent. The diagnosis of a glaucoma suspect is also dependent on a normal open angle on gonioscopy.

The most common finding warranting this diagnosis is elevated IOP in the absence of identifiable optic nerve damage or visual field loss, a condition often termed *ocular hypertension.* Estimates of the prevalence of ocular hypertension vary considerably; some authorities believe it may be as high as eight times that of definite POAG. Analysis of studies that have followed individuals with elevated IOP for variable time periods indicates that the higher the baseline IOP, the greater the risk of developing glaucoma. However, it is important to note that even among individuals with elevated IOP, the vast majority never develop glaucoma.

Differentiating between a diagnosis of ocular hypertension versus early primary open-angle glaucoma is often difficult. The ophthalmologist must look carefully for signs of early damage to the optic nerve, such as focal notching, asymmetry of cupping, splinter disc hemorrhage, nerve fiber layer dropout, or subtle visual field defects. The increasing use of shortwave and frequency doubling automated perimetry may improve our ability to recognize early glaucomatous visual field loss in these patients (see chapter III). If these signs of optic nerve damage are present, the diagnosis of early POAG should be considered and treatment initiated. However, an ophthalmologist should not be hesitant about monitoring closely a patient off therapy to document progressive changes or confirm the present findings in order to better establish the diagnosis prior to initiating therapy.

No clear consensus exists on whether elevated IOP should be treated in the absence of signs of early damage. Some ophthalmologists treat all individuals with elevated IOP, especially when it exceeds 30 mm Hg, while others do not treat without evidence of some optic nerve damage or early visual field loss. Some clinicians select and treat those individuals thought to be at greatest risk for developing glaucoma after assessing all risk factors.

All available data must be weighed in assessing the patient's risk for developing glaucoma and deciding whether to treat elevated IOP. The following risk factors should be considered:

□ Level of elevated IOP

□ Family history of glaucoma

□ Race

□ Age

□ Associated disease states (diabetes mellitus, systemic hypertension, and cardiovascular disease)

Most ophthalmologists initiate treatment if the IOP is consistently higher than 30 mm Hg, because of the high risk of optic disc damage. If the clinician elects to treat solely on the basis of IOP, care must be taken that the risks of therapy do not exceed the risk of the disease. The target IOP in patients without demonstrated damage to the optic nerve can be somewhat flexible. Additional factors that may affect the decision to start ocular hypertensive therapy include the desires of the patient, compliance, availability for follow-up visits, corneal pachymetry, reliability of visual fields, and ability to examine the optic disc.

An ongoing multicenter randomized clinical trial sponsored by the National Eye Institute, the Ocular Hypertension Treatment Study, is addressing the question of the effect of medical treatment compared with observation of individuals with elevated IOP but no signs of glaucoma (see Table IV-2). This study should also help identify what characteristics or combinations of characteristics place individuals at increased risk of developing optic nerve damage.

Preferred Practice Patterns Committee, Glaucoma Panel. *The Glaucoma Suspect.* San Francisco: American Academy of Ophthalmology; 2000.

## Normal-Tension Glaucoma

Considerable controversy remains about whether normal-tension glaucoma represents a distinct disease entity or is simply primary open-angle glaucoma with IOP within the normal range. Because IOP is a continuous variable with no firm dividing line between normal and abnormal, many authorities believe the terms *low-tension* and *normal-tension glaucoma* should be abandoned. This debate is likely to persist. Whatever the outcome, the concept of normal-tension glaucoma has undeniably had a strong influence on the classification and understanding of glaucoma.

### Clinical Features

As previously emphasized, elevated IOP is an important risk factor in the development of glaucoma, but it is not the only risk factor. In normal-tension glaucoma other risk factors, most of which are currently unknown, may play a more important role. Many authorities have hypothesized that local vascular factors may have a significant part in the development of this disorder. Studies have suggested that patients with normal-tension glaucoma show a higher prevalence of vasospastic disorders such as migraine headache and Raynaud phenomenon, ischemic vascular diseases, autoimmune diseases, and coagulopathies compared with patients who have high-tension glaucoma. However, these findings have not been consistent. Vascular autoregulatory defects have also been described in studies of eyes with normal-tension glaucoma.

Field loss consistent with glaucoma has been noted after a decrease in blood pressure following a hypotensive crisis. However, damage secondary to such a specific precipitating event tends to be stable and does not progress once the underlying problem has been corrected. Most cases of normal-tension glaucoma are not caused by a sudden precipitating event. The condition is characteristically progressive, often despite the lowering of IOP. The association between IOP and normal-tension glaucoma has long been controversial. Studies have indicated that in glaucomatous eyes with normal but asymmetric IOP, the worse damage usually occurs in the eye with the higher IOP. The Collaborative Normal-Tension Glaucoma Study found that reducing IOP by greater than 30% reduced the rate of visual field progression from 35% to 12%, confirming a clear role of IOP in this disease. However, since progression was not affected in all patients, other factors may be operative as well. In addition, progression of the visual field loss, when it did occur, tended to be slow.

> Collaborative Normal-Tension Glaucoma Study Group. Comparison of glaucomatous progression between untreated patients with normal-tension glaucoma and patients with therapeutically reduced intraocular pressures. *Am J Ophthalmol.* 1998;126: 487–497.

Another area of considerable debate concerns patterns of optic disc damage and visual field loss in normal-tension compared with primary open-angle glaucoma. In eyes matched for total visual field loss, the neuroretinal rim has been reported to be thinner, especially inferiorly and inferotemporally, in those with normal-tension glaucoma. Varied patterns of peripapillary atrophy may also be characteristic for normal-tension glaucoma. Some authorities have separated normal-tension glaucoma into two forms based on disc appearance:

- A *senile sclerotic group* with shallow, pale sloping of the neuroretinal rim (primarily in older patients with vascular disease)
- A *focal ischemic group* with deep, focal, polar notching in the neuroretinal rim

The visual field defects in normal-tension glaucoma tend to be more focal, deeper, and closer to fixation, especially early in the course of the disease, compared with what is commonly seen in primary open-angle glaucoma. A dense paracentral scotoma encroaching on fixation is not an unusual finding as the initial defect. The validity of many of the reports of purported differences between normal-tension and primary open-angle glaucoma has been disputed, however, by other studies that have found no differences in these characteristics.

## Differential Diagnosis

Normal-tension glaucoma can be mimicked by many conditions:

- Vascular occlusion
- Optic nerve head drusen
- Optic nerve head pits and colobomas
- Chorioretinitis
- Retinal detachment
- Retinoschisis
- Chiasmal tumors
- Anterior ischemic optic neuropathy

Several of these conditions can cause arcuate-type visual field defects.

Care must be taken to distinguish normal-tension glaucoma from undetected primary open-angle glaucoma, secondary open-angle glaucoma such as pigmentary glaucoma, and nonglaucomatous optic nerve disease (Table IV-4). Diurnal IOP measurement is critical to determine with confidence that glaucomatous damage is occurring with IOPs consistently in the normal range.

Elevated IOP can be obscured in patients taking systemic medication, particularly systemic beta blockers, and by artifactually low tonometric readings caused, for example, by reduced scleral rigidity and corneal thickness following refractive surgery. Assessment of central corneal thickness is recommended in patients suspected of having normal-tension glaucoma. Other conditions to consider in the differential diagnosis include normalized IOP in an eye with previously elevated IOP, intermittent angle-closure glaucoma, and previous corticosteroid-induced or other secondary glaucoma.

## Diagnostic Evaluation

It is difficult to know how often glaucomatous damage occurs with IOP in the normal range. Population-based epidemiologic studies have suggested that as many as 30%–50% of glaucomatous eyes may have IOP below 21 mm Hg on a single reading. Repeated testing would undoubtedly have detected elevated IOP in many of these eyes. The prevalence of normal-tension glaucoma appears to vary among different populations. Studies have suggested that among Japanese patients a particularly high proportion of open-angle glaucoma occurs with IOP in the normal range. Among clinic-based patients a diagnosis of normal-tension glaucoma is influenced by how thoroughly other possible causes of optic neuropathy are considered and eliminated.

TABLE IV-4

DIFFERENTIAL DIAGNOSIS OF NORMAL-TENSION GLAUCOMA

**Undetected high-tension glaucoma**

Primary open-angle glaucoma with diurnal IOP variation

Intermittent IOP elevation
  Angle-closure glaucoma
  Glaucomatocyclitic crisis

Previously elevated IOP
  Old secondary glaucoma (e.g., corticosteroid-induced glaucoma, uveitic glaucoma, pigmentary glaucoma)
  Normalized IOP in an eye with previously elevated IOP

Use of medication that may cause IOP lowering (systemic beta blocker)

Tonometric error (reduced corneal thickness, low scleral rigidity)

**Nonglaucomatous optic nerve disease**

Congenital anomalies (coloboma, optic nerve pits)

Compressive lesions of optic nerve and chiasm

Shock optic neuropathy

Anterior ischemic optic neuropathy

Retinal disorders (i.e., retinal detachment, retinoschisis)

Optic nerve drusen

Before making a diagnosis of normal-tension glaucoma, the clinician should measure the patient's IOP by applanation tonometry at various times during the day. Gonioscopy should be performed to rule out angle closure, angle recession, or evidence of previous intraocular inflammation. Careful stereoscopic disc evaluation is essential to rule out other congenital or acquired disc anomalies, such as optic nerve coloboma or drusen. The clinician must also consider the patient's medical history, particularly any record of cardiovascular disease and low blood pressure caused by hemorrhage, myocardial infarction, or shock.

Sometimes a diagnosis cannot be established on the basis of a single or even multiple ophthalmic examinations, particularly if findings are atypical, as in unilateral disease, decreased central vision, or visual field loss not consistent with the optic disc appearance. In such cases medical and neurologic evaluation should be considered, including tests for anemia, heart disease, syphilis, and temporal arteritis or other causes of systemic vasculitis. Auscultation and palpation of the carotid arteries should be performed, and noninvasive tests of carotid circulation may be helpful. Increasing attention is being focused on assessment of ocular blood flow, but techniques for these measurements are generally still investigational. Evaluation of the optic nerve in the chiasmal region with computed tomography (CT) or magnetic resonance imaging (MRI) may be warranted in some cases to rule out compressive lesions, especially if the visual field loss is at all suggestive of congruous, bitemporal, or other neurologic defects (see also BCSC Section 5, *Neuro-Ophthalmology*).

## Prognosis and Therapy

Therapy for normal-tension glaucoma can be difficult and controversial. It is generally initiated for normal-tension glaucoma unless the optic neuropathy is determined to be stable. The results of the Collaborative Normal-Tension Glaucoma Study support aggressive reduction in IOP by greater than 30% in an attempt to reduce progressive visual field loss. The criteria for initiating therapy in this study were visual field loss threatening fixation, disc hemorrhage, and documented visual field or optic nerve progression. This study demonstrated that disease in some patients (65%) did not progress over the length of the study despite the lack of treatment, while in others (12%) it did progress despite aggressive reduction in IOP, demonstrating the extremely variable clinical course. The role of "neuroprotective" agents such as calcium channel blockers, alpha$_2$-adrenergic agonists, and NMDA (N-methyl-D-aspartate receptor) antagonists is experimental and highly controversial (see chapter VII). The goal of therapy should be to achieve an IOP as low as possible without inducing complications using the knowledge currently available.

Systemic medications such as calcium channel blockers are advocated by some authorities because of the possible beneficial effects of increasing capillary perfusion of the optic nerve head. The efficacy of this treatment, however, has not been demonstrated. If systemic treatment with calcium channel blockers is undertaken, it should be coordinated with the patient's primary care physician because of possible side effects. Systemic hypotension, a possible complication of this therapy, may adversely affect ocular blood flow.

As with POAG, medical therapy is the most common initial approach in treating normal-tension glaucoma. As with all glaucomas, it is useful for the ophthalmologist to change or add medications to one eye at a time, so that the contralateral eye can be used as a control to assess therapeutic response. If medications are inadequate in controlling the disease, laser trabeculoplasty can be effective in reducing IOP. Glaucoma filtering surgery may be indicated in an attempt to obtain the lowest IOP. An antifibrotic agent, 5-fluorouracil or mitomycin-C, may be used to improve the success rate of filtering surgery and to reduce the postoperative and long-term IOP (see chapter VIII).

Bhandari A, Crabb DP, Poinoosawny D, et al. Effect of surgery on visual field progression in normal-tension glaucoma. *Ophthalmology.* 1997;104:1131–1137.

Collaborative Normal-Tension Glaucoma Study Group. The effectiveness of intraocular pressure reduction in the treatment of normal-tension glaucoma. *Am J Ophthalmol.* 1998;126:498–505.

Collaborative Normal-Tension Glaucoma Study Group. Comparison of glaucomatous progression between untreated patients with normal-tension glaucoma and patients with therapeutically reduced intraocular pressures. *Am J Ophthalmol.* 1998;126:487–497.

## Secondary Open-Angle Glaucoma

### Exfoliation Syndrome (Pseudoexfoliation)

*Exfoliation syndrome* is characterized by the deposition of a distinctive fibrillar material in the anterior segment of the eye. Histologically, this material has been found in and on the lens epithelium and capsule, pupillary margin, ciliary epithelium, iris pigment epithelium, iris stroma and blood vessels, and subconjunctival tissue. Although the origin of this material is not known precisely, it probably arises from

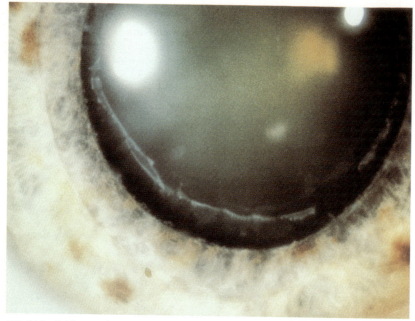

FIG IV-1—Evidence of exfoliative material deposited on the anterior lens capsule. Exfoliative material may also be deposited on other structures within the anterior segment, including the iris, ciliary processes, peripheral retina, and the conjunctiva.

multiple sources as part of a generalized basement membrane disorder. Histochemically, the material resembles amyloid.

Deposits occur in a targetlike pattern on the anterior lens capsule and are best seen after pupil dilation. A central area and a peripheral zone of deposition are usually separated by an intermediate clear area, where iris movement presumably rubs the material from the lens (Fig IV-1). The material is often visible on the iris at the edge of the pupil. Deposits also occur on the zonular fibers of the lens, ciliary processes, inferior anterior chamber angle, and corneal endothelium (Fig IV-2). In aphakic individuals these deposits may be seen on the anterior hyaloid as well.

The chamber angle is often characterized by a trabecular meshwork that is heavily pigmented (with dark, almost black pigment), usually in a variegated fashion. An inferior pigmented deposition, scalloped in nature, is often present anterior to Schwalbe's line (Sampoelesi's line, Fig IV-3). The chamber angle is often shallow, presumably as a result of anterior movement of the lens–iris diaphragm related to zonular weakness.

In addition to the typical deposits and pigmentation, other anterior segment abnormalities are also noted. Fine pigment deposits often appear on the iris surface, and peripupillary atrophy with transillumination of the pupillary margin is common. A more scattered, diffuse depigmentation may also occur, with transillumination defect over the entire sphincter region. Phacodonesis and iridodonesis are not uncommon, and they are most likely related to zonular weakness, which may pre-

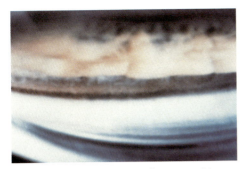

FIG IV-2—Exfoliative debris collecting on iris processes in inferior anterior chamber angle.

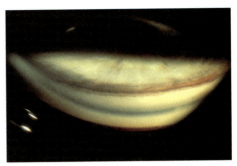

FIG IV-3—Sampoelesi's line in the inferior anterior chamber angle of a patient who has exfoliation syndrome. (Photograph courtesy of L.J. Katz, MD.)

dispose affected eyes to zonular dehiscence, vitreous loss, and other complications during cataract surgery (see also BCSC Section 11, *Lens and Cataract*). Iris angiography has demonstrated abnormalities of the iris vessels through fluorescein leakage.

Exfoliation syndrome may be monocular or binocular with varying degrees of asymmetry. Often the disorder is clinically apparent in only one eye, although the uninvolved fellow eye may develop the syndrome at a later time. Exfoliation syndrome is associated with open-angle glaucoma in all populations, but the prevalence varies considerably. In Scandinavian countries exfoliation syndrome accounts for more than 50% of cases of open-angle glaucoma. This syndrome is strongly age-related: it is rarely seen under the age of 50 and occurs most commonly in individuals over the age of 70.

The open-angle glaucoma associated with exfoliation syndrome is thought to be caused by the fibrillar material obstructing flow through and causing damage to the trabecular meshwork. Exfoliation syndrome with glaucoma differs from primary open-angle glaucoma in often being monocular and showing greater pigmentation of the trabecular meshwork. Furthermore, the IOP is often higher than it is in primary open-angle glaucoma, and the overall prognosis is worse. Laser trabeculoplasty can be very effective, but the response may not be long lasting, and lens extraction does not alleviate the condition. Trabeculectomy results are similar to those with primary open-angle glaucoma, but there may be an increase in postoperative inflammation. In fact, increased ocular inflammation can be seen following all ocular surgery in patients with this condition.

## Pigmentary Glaucoma

The *pigment dispersion syndrome* consists of pigment deposition on the corneal endothelium in a vertical spindle pattern (Krukenberg spindle), in the trabecular meshwork, and on the lens periphery (Fig IV-4). The spindle pattern on the posterior cornea is caused by the aqueous convection currents and subsequent phagocytosis of pigment by the corneal endothelium. The presence of Krukenberg spindles is not absolutely necessary to make the diagnosis of pigment dispersion syndrome, and it may occur in other diseases such as exfoliation syndrome. Characteristic spokelike

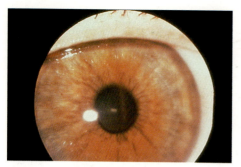

FIG IV-4—Krukenberg spindle. (Photograph courtesy of L.J. Katz, MD.)

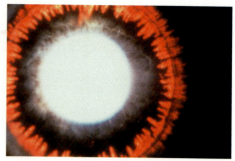

FIG IV-5—Classic spokelike iris transillumination defects seen in pigmentary dispersion syndrome. (Photograph courtesy of L.J. Katz, MD.)

loss of the iris pigment epithelium occurs that is manifested as transillumination defects in the iris midperiphery (Fig IV-5). The peripheral iris transillumination defects appear in front of the lens zonular fibers, confirming that mechanical contact between the zonular packets and the iris contributes to the iris pigment release.

Gonioscopy reveals a homogeneous, densely pigmented trabecular meshwork with a speckled ring of pigment at or anterior to Schwalbe's line (Fig IV-6). The midperipheral iris is often concave in appearance, bowing posterior toward the lens zonules. When dilated, pigment deposits can be seen on the lens zonules and both the anterior and posterior lens capsule (Fig IV-7).

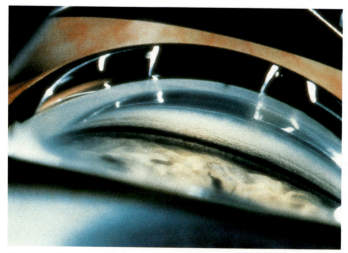

FIG IV-6—Characteristic heavy, uniform pigmentation of the trabecular meshwork seen in the pigment dispersion syndrome and pigmentary glaucoma.

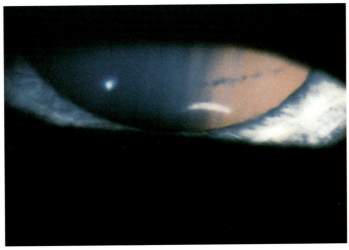

FIG IV-7—In pigmentary dispersion syndrome, pigment deposits can be seen on the anterior and posterior lens capsule and on the lens zonules with gonioscopy in dilated eye.

This syndrome may or may not be associated with glaucoma. An individual with pigment dispersion syndrome may never develop elevated IOP, and various studies have suggested that the risk of an affected individual developing glaucoma is approximately 25%–50%. Pigmentary glaucoma occurs most commonly in myopic males between the ages of 20 and 50 years. Affected females tend to be older than affected males.

Pigmentary glaucoma is characterized by wide fluctuations in IOP, which can exceed 50 mm Hg in the untreated patient. High IOP often occurs when pigment is released into the aqueous humor, such as following exercise or pupillary dilation. Symptoms may include haloes, intermittent visual blurring, and ocular pain. Medical treatment is often successful in reducing IOP. Patients respond reasonably well to laser trabeculoplasty, although the effect may be short-lived. Filtering surgery is usually successful.

Posterior bowing of the iris with "reverse pupillary block" configuration is noted in many eyes that have pigmentary glaucoma. This iris configuration may result in greater contact of the zonular fibers with the posterior iris surface, with a subsequent increase of pigment release. Laser iridectomy has been proposed as a means of minimizing posterior bowing of the iris (Fig IV-8). However, its effectiveness for the treatment of pigmentary glaucoma has not been established. Currently, laser iridectomy is most often applied in eyes with pigment dispersion and ocular hypertension or early glaucomatous optic neuropathy.

With age the signs and symptoms of pigmentary dispersion may decrease in some individuals, possibly as a result of normal growth of the lens and an increase in physiologic pupillary block. Loss of accommodation may also be a factor.

Liebmann JM. Pigmentary glaucoma: new insights. In: *Focal Points: Clinical Modules for Ophthalmologists.* San Francisco: American Academy of Ophthalmology; 1998: vol 16, no 2.

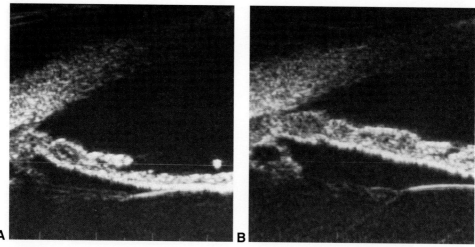

FIG IV-8—*A,* Ultrasound biomicroscopy image of concave iris configuration in pigmentary glaucoma, pre–laser treatment. *B,* Same eye, post–laser treatment. (Photographs courtesy of Charles J. Pavlin, MD.)

### Lens-Induced Glaucoma

The lens may cause both open-angle and angle-closure glaucomas, and these are summarized in Table IV-5. The open-angle lens-induced glaucomas are divided into three clinical entities:

□ Phacolytic glaucoma

□ Lens particle glaucoma

□ Phacoanaphylaxis

See also BCSC Section 9, *Intraocular Inflammation and Uveitis,* and Section 11, *Lens and Cataract.*

***Phacolytic glaucoma*** This inflammatory glaucoma is caused by the leakage of lens protein through the capsule of a mature or hypermature cataract (Fig IV-9). As the lens ages, its protein composition becomes altered, with an increased concentration

TABLE IV-5

LENS-INDUCED GLAUCOMAS

| **Open-angle** | **Angle-closure** (see chapter V) |
|---|---|
| Phacolytic glaucoma | Phacomorphic |
| Lens particle glaucoma | Ectopia lentis |
| Phacoanaphylaxis | |

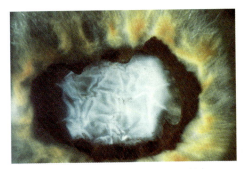 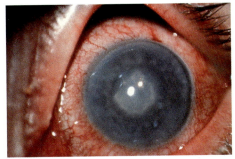

FIG IV-9—Characteristic appearance of hypermature cataract with loss of cortical volume and wrinkling of the anterior lens capsule. Extensive posterior synechiae are present, confirming the presence of previous inflammation.

FIG IV-10—Phacolytic glaucoma. Conjunctival hyperemia, microcystic corneal edema, mature cataract, and prominent anterior chamber reaction without keratic precipitates is the typical presentation of phacolytic glaucoma, as demonstrated in this photograph. (Photograph courtesy of the Wills Eye Hospital slide collection, 1986.)

of high-molecular-weight lens protein. In a mature or hypermature cataract these proteins are released through microscopic openings in the lens capsule. The proteins precipitate an inflammatory reaction that causes a secondary glaucoma, as lens material–filled macrophages and other inflammatory debris obstruct the trabecular meshwork.

The clinical picture usually involves an elderly patient with a history of poor vision who has sudden onset of pain, conjunctival hyperemia, and worsening vision. Examination reveals an elevated IOP of 30–50 mm Hg, microcystic corneal edema, a prominent cell and flare reaction without keratic precipitates (KP), and an open anterior chamber angle (Fig IV-10). The lack of KP helps distinguish phacolytic glaucoma from phacoanaphylaxis. Cellular debris may be seen layering in the anterior chamber angle, and a hypopyon may be present. White particles (clumps of lens protein) may also be seen in the anterior chamber. A mature, hypermature, or morgagnian cataract is present, often with wrinkling of the anterior lens capsule representing loss of volume and the release of lens material (see Figure IV-9). While medications to control the IOP should be used immediately, definitive therapy requires cataract extraction.

***Lens particle glaucoma*** This glaucoma occurs when the lens cortex obstructs the trabecular meshwork following cataract extraction, capsulotomy, or ocular trauma. The extent of the glaucoma depends on the quantity of lens material released, the extent of inflammatory response, the preexisting ability of the trabecular meshwork to clear the lens material, and the functional status of the ciliary body, which is often altered following surgery or trauma.

Lens particle glaucoma usually occurs within weeks of the initial surgery or trauma, but it may occur months or years later (Figs IV-11, IV-12). Clinical findings include free cortical material in the anterior chamber, elevated IOP, moderate anterior chamber reaction, microcystic corneal edema, and, with time, the development of posterior and peripheral anterior synechiae.

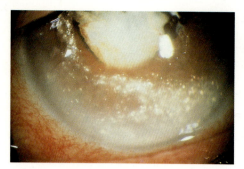

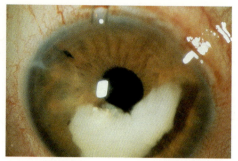

FIG IV-11—Lens particle glaucoma. Cortical lens material obstructs the trabecular meshwork following traumatic disruption of the anterior lens capsule.

FIG IV-12—Lens particle glaucoma. Despite the large amount of lens cortex remaining in the anterior chamber following cataract surgery, this eye is relatively quiet and the IOP remained normal. (Photograph courtesy of the Wills Eye Hospital slide collection, 1986.)

If possible, medical therapy should be initiated to control the IOP while the residual lens material resorbs. Appropriate therapy includes medications to decrease aqueous formation, mydriatics to inhibit posterior synechiae formation, and topical corticosteroids to reduce inflammation. If the glaucoma cannot be controlled, surgical removal of the lens material is necessary.

**Phacoanaphylaxis**  Phacoanaphylaxis is a rare entity in which patients become sensitized to their own lens protein following surgery or penetrating trauma, resulting in a granulomatous inflammation. The clinical picture is quite variable, but most patients present with a moderate anterior chamber reaction with KP on both the corneal endothelium and the anterior lens surface. In addition, a low-grade vitritis, synechial formation, and residual lens material in the anterior chamber may be found. Phacoanaphylaxis is treated medically with corticosteroids and aqueous suppressants to reduce inflammation and IOP. If medical treatment is unsuccessful, residual lens material should be removed. Glaucoma, while it may occur, is not common in eyes with phacoanaphylaxis.

## Intraocular Tumors

A variety of tumors can cause unilateral chronic glaucoma. Many of the tumors described below are discussed in greater detail in BCSC Section 4, *Ophthalmic Pathology and Intraocular Tumors*. Variation in the location, type, and size of the tumor means the glaucoma can result from several different mechanisms:

□ Direct tumor invasion of the anterior chamber angle

□ Angle closure by rotation of the ciliary body or by anterior displacement of the lens–iris diaphragm (see chapter V)

□ Intraocular hemorrhage

□ Neovascularization of the angle

□ Deposition of tumor cells, inflammatory cells, and cellular debris within the trabecular meshwork

Choroidal melanomas and other choroidal and retinal tumors tend to cause secondary angle-closure glaucoma as the result of a forward shift in the lens–iris diaphragm and closure of the anterior chamber angle. Inflammation caused by necrotic tumors may cause posterior synechiae, which can exacerbate this angle closure through a pupillary-block mechanism. Choroidal melanomas, medulloepitheliomas, and retinoblastomas can also cause anterior segment neovascularization, which can result in angle closure.

The most common cause of glaucoma in primary or metastatic tumors of the ciliary body is direct angle invasion. This glaucoma can be exacerbated by anterior segment hemorrhage and inflammation, which further obstruct outflow. Necrotic tumor and tumor-filled macrophages may cause obstruction of the trabecular meshwork and result in a secondary open-angle glaucoma. Tumors causing glaucoma in adults include uveal melanoma, metastatic carcinoma, lymphomas, and leukemia. Glaucoma in children is associated with retinoblastoma, juvenile xanthogranuloma, and medulloepithelioma.

## Ocular Inflammation and Secondary Open-Angle Glaucoma

Inflammatory glaucoma is a secondary glaucoma that often combines components of open-angle and angle-closure disease and occurs when the trabecular dysfunction exceeds the accompanying ciliary body hyposecretion seen with acute inflammation. Often the ocular inflammation is nonspecific. When the inflammation is accompanied by increased IOP, the physician's dilemma is whether the cause of the increased IOP is the active inflammation and insufficient anti-inflammatory therapy or chronic structural damage related to the underlying inflammation or to corticosteroid therapy.

Open-angle inflammatory glaucoma is caused by a variety of mechanisms:

□ Edema of the trabecular meshwork

□ Endothelial cell dysfunction

□ Blockage of the trabecular meshwork by fibrin and inflammatory cells

□ Prostaglandin-mediated breakdown of the blood–aqueous barrier

Most of the causes of anterior uveitis are unknown, but herpes zoster iridocyclitis, herpes simplex keratouveitis, toxoplasmosis, rheumatoid arthritis, and pars planitis are common causes of open-angle inflammatory glaucoma. See also BCSC Section 9, *Intraocular Inflammation and Uveitis.*

The presence of keratic precipitates and a miotic pupil suggests *iritis* as the cause of IOP elevation. Gonioscopic evaluation may reveal subtle trabecular meshwork precipitates. Sometimes, PAS or posterior synechiae with iris bombé may develop, resulting in angle closure. The treatment of inflammatory glaucoma is complicated by the fact that corticosteroid therapy may raise IOP, either by reducing inflammation and improving aqueous production or by decreasing outflow. Miotic agents should be avoided in patients with iritis, because they may aggravate the inflammation and cause posterior synechiae.

***Glaucomatocyclitic crisis (Posner-Schlossman syndrome)*** This form of open-angle inflammatory glaucoma is characterized by recurrent bouts of markedly increased IOP and low-grade anterior chamber inflammation. First described by Posner and Schlossman in 1948, the condition affects middle-aged patients and usually presents with unilateral blurred vision and mild eye pain. The iritis is mild with few KP that are small, discreet, and round in nature and usually resolve spontaneously within a few weeks. KP may be seen on the trabecular meshwork on gonioscopy, suggesting a "trabeculitis." The IOP is usually markedly elevated, in the 40–50 mm Hg range, and corneal edema may be present. In between bouts the IOP usually returns to normal, but, with increasing numbers of attacks, a chronic secondary glaucoma may develop. The etiology of the disease remains unknown, but a prostaglandin-mediated mechanism has been proposed.

***Fuchs heterochromic iridocyclitis*** This relatively rare, chronic form of iridocyclitis is characterized by iris heterochromia (with loss of iris pigment in the affected eye); low-grade anterior chamber reaction with small, stellate KP; posterior subcapsular cataracts; and secondary open-angle glaucoma. The condition is insidious and unilateral, affecting the hypochromic eye, and presents equally in middle-aged men and women. The secondary open-angle glaucoma occurs in approximately 15% of the cases, also in middle-aged men and women. Gonioscopy reveals multiple fine vessels that cross the trabecular meshwork (Fig IV-13). These vessels, unlike those in iris neovascularization, do not appear to be associated with a fibrous membrane and usually do not lead to PAS and secondary angle closure. These vessels are fragile and may cause an anterior chamber hemorrhage, either spontaneously or with trauma (Fig IV-14).

The glaucoma does not correspond to the degree of inflammation and may be difficult to control. Corticosteroids are generally not effective in treating this condition. Aqueous suppressants and alpha$_2$-adrenergic agonists are the agents of choice.

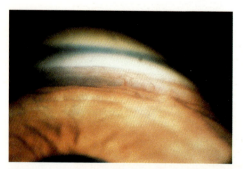 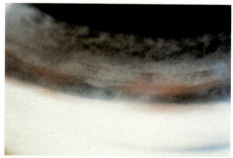

FIG IV-13—Fuchs heterochromic iridocyclitis. Fine vessels are seen crossing the trabecular meshwork. This neovascularization is not accompanied by a fibrovascular membrane and does not result in peripheral anterior synechiae formation and secondary angle closure.

FIG IV-14—The atypical vessels seen in the anterior chamber angle of patients with Fuchs heterochromic iridocyclitis are fragile and can result in a filiform hemorrhage. This hemorrhage often occurs spontaneously or with minimal trauma, as demonstrated in this photograph.

TABLE IV-6

CAUSES OF INCREASED EPISCLERAL PRESSURE

**Arteriovenous malformations**
    Arteriovenous fistula (carotid–dural)
    Orbital varix
    Sturge-Weber syndrome

**Venous obstruction**
    Retrobulbar tumor
    Thyroid ophthalmopathy

**Superior vena cava syndrome**

## Raised Episcleral Venous Pressure

Episcleral venous pressure is an important factor in the regulation of IOP. Normal episcleral venous pressure is approximately 9 mm Hg, but it can be raised by a variety of clinical entities that either obstruct venous outflow or involve arteriovenous malformations. A partial list of entities that increase episcleral venous pressure is presented in Table IV-6.

Clinically, patients with increased episcleral venous pressure present with tortuous, dilated episcleral veins (Fig IV-15). These vascular changes may be unilateral or bilateral depending on the location of the vascular anomaly. The anterior segment appears normal in most of these patients, except for elevated IOP and the gonioscopic finding of blood in Schlemm's canal. Rarely, signs of ocular ischemia or venous stasis may be present.

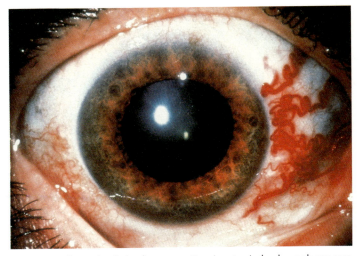

FIG IV-15—Elevated episcleral pressure. Prominent episcleral vessels are seen in a patient with Sturge-Weber syndrome. Patients with increased episcleral pressure present with tortuous, dilated episcleral vessels.

Medications that reduce aqueous humor formation are more effective than drugs that increase aqueous outflow. Laser trabeculoplasty is not effective unless there are secondary changes in the outflow channels. Glaucoma filtering surgery may be complicated by ciliochoroidal effusions or suprachoroidal hemorrhage.

## Accidental and Surgical Trauma

Nonpenetrating, or blunt, trauma to the eye causes a variety of anterior segment injuries:

- Hyphema
- Angle recession (cleavage)
- Iridodialysis
- Iris sphincter tear
- Cyclodialysis
- Lens subluxation

A combination of posttraumatic inflammation, presence of blood and degenerative red blood cells (ghost cells), and direct injury to the trabecular meshwork often results in elevated IOP initially after trauma. This elevation tends to be short in duration but may be protracted with the risk of corneal blood staining (Fig IV-16) and glaucomatous optic nerve damage.

Patients with *sickle cell disease* pose a therapeutic dilemma because the acidic environment of the anterior chamber promotes sickling, which impedes the egress of red blood cells through the trabecular meshwork as a result of their reduced pliability. Once sickling occurs, the eye is more prone to increased IOP and more susceptible to associated ischemic complications such as anterior ischemic optic neuropathy and central retinal artery occlusion.

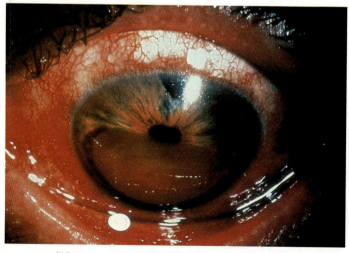

FIG IV-16—Corneal blood staining following trauma.

Open-angle glaucoma is one of the long-term sequelae of *siderosis* or *chalcosis* from a retained intraocular metallic foreign body in penetrating or perforating injuries. Chemical injuries, particularly alkali, may cause acute secondary glaucoma as a result of inflammation, shrinkage of scleral collagen, release of chemical mediators such as prostaglandins, direct damage to the chamber angle, or compromise of the anterior uveal circulation. Trabecular damage or inflammation may cause glaucoma to develop months or years after a chemical injury.

***Traumatic, or angle-recession, glaucoma***   An angle recession, or cleavage, is a tear in the ciliary body that splits between the longitudinal and circular muscle fibers. Angle recessions are often associated with tears in the trabecular meshwork as well. Angle-recession glaucoma is a chronic, unilateral secondary open-angle glaucoma that usually occurs months to years following ocular trauma. It resembles primary open-angle glaucoma in presentation and clinical course but can usually be distinguished by its classic gonioscopic findings (Figs IV-17, IV-18):

□ Broad angle recess

□ Absent or torn iris processes

□ White glistening scleral spur

□ Depression in the overlying trabecular meshwork

□ Localized PAS at the border of the recession

The degree of angle involvement and underlying patient predisposition play an important role in determining whether a secondary glaucoma will develop. A significant proportion (up to 50%) of fellow eyes may develop increased IOP, suggesting that perhaps many eyes with angle-recession glaucoma may have been predisposed to open-angle glaucoma.

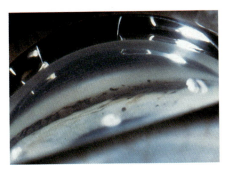

FIG IV-17—An angle recession occurs when the ciliary body is torn between the longitudinal and circular fibers of the ciliary body. There is a deepened angle recess as a result of atrophy of the circular fibers. (Photograph courtesy of Joseph Krug, MD.)

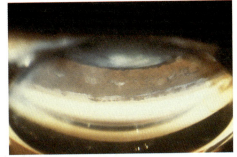

FIG IV-18—Typical angle appearance of an angle recession. Torn iris processes; a whitened, increasingly visible scleral spur; and a localized depression of the trabecular meshwork are seen.

The greater the extent of the angle recession, the greater the risk of glaucoma. Even with substantial angle recession, this risk is not high, but all eyes with angle recession must be followed closely because it is not possible to predict which eyes will develop glaucoma. Although the risk of developing glaucoma decreases appreciably after several years, the risk is still present even 20–25 years following injury, and these eyes should continue to be examined annually.

The treatment of angle-recession glaucoma is best accomplished with aqueous suppressants and alpha$_2$-adrenergic agonists. Miotics may be useful, but paradoxical responses with increased IOP may occur. The role of prostaglandin analogues has not been studied. Laser trabeculoplasty has a limited role and a low chance of success but may be considered prior to filtering surgery.

***Cyclodialysis cleft*** Glaucoma may also result from closure of a cyclodialysis cleft. In contrast to angle recession, histopathologic examination of a cyclodialysis cleft shows a focal area of separation of the ciliary body from its attachment to the scleral spur. When a cyclodialysis cleft is present, the eye is often hypotonous. The mechanism of the hypotony is thought to be related to increased uveoscleral outflow through the cleft into suprachoroidal space and possibly reduced aqueous production as a result of vascular compromise to the ciliary processes. If the cleft closes, the IOP may become quite elevated. The trabecular meshwork function may improve spontaneously with time, requiring only temporary treatment of the IOP. Occasionally, long-term elevation of IOP persists, and this condition is treated in a manner similar to primary open-angle glaucoma.

***Hyphema*** Glaucoma may result from hyphema through several mechanisms (Fig IV-19). Increased IOP is more common following recurrent hemorrhage or rebleeding following a traumatic hyphema. The reported frequency of rebleeding following hyphema varies considerably in the literature, with an average incidence of 5%–10%. Rebleeding usually occurs within 5–7 days after the initial hyphema and may be related to normal clot retraction and lysis. In most cases the size of the hyphema associated with rebleeding is greater than the primary hyphema. In general, the larger the hyphema, the higher the incidence of increased IOP, although small hemorrhages may also be associated with marked elevation of IOP, especially in the already compromised angle. Increased IOP is a result of obstruction of the trabecular meshwork with red blood cells, inflammatory cells, debris, and fibrin, and direct injury to the trabecular meshwork from the blunt trauma.

Individuals with *sickle cell hemoglobinopathies* have an increased incidence of glaucoma following hyphema. Normal red blood cells generally pass through the trabecular meshwork without difficulty. However, in the sickle cell hemoglobinopathies (including sickle trait), the red blood cells tend to sickle in the aqueous humor, and these more rigid cells have great difficulty passing out of the eye through the trabecular meshwork. Even small amounts of blood in the anterior chamber may therefore result in marked elevations of IOP. In addition, the optic discs of patients with sickle cell disease are much more sensitive to elevated IOP and are prone to ischemic injury as a result of compromised microvascular perfusion.

In general, an uncomplicated hyphema should be managed conservatively with an eyeshield, limited activity, and head elevation. Topical and systemic corticosteroids may reduce associated inflammation, although their effect on rebleeding is debatable. If significant ciliary spasm or photophobia occurs, cycloplegic agents

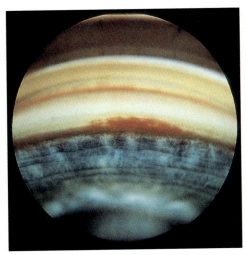

FIG IV-19—A small hyphema seen gonioscopically in the inferior chamber angle with layering of blood on the trabecular meshwork.

may be helpful, but they have no proven benefit in terms of rebleeding. Amino-caproic acid has been shown to reduce rebleeding, but reports on its efficacy and associated complications are conflicting. Patching and bed rest are also advocated by some authors, although these precautions are of unproven value.

If the IOP is elevated, aqueous suppressants, alpha$_2$-adrenergic agonists, and hyperosmotic agents are recommended. It has been suggested that patients with sickle cell hemoglobinopathies should avoid carbonic anhydrase inhibitors, as they may increase the sickling tendency in the anterior chamber by increasing aqueous levels of ascorbic acid; however, this relationship has not been firmly established. Adrenergic agonists with significant alpha$_1$ effects (apraclonidine, dipivefrin, epinephrine) should also be avoided in sickle cell disease. Parasympathomimetic agents should be avoided in all patients with hyphemas.

Persistently elevated IOP may require surgery. The potential of inducing amblyopia if the hyphema is significantly obstructing vision may justify early surgical intervention in very young children. If surgery for increased IOP becomes necessary, an anterior chamber irrigation or washout procedure is commonly tried first. If a total hyphema is present, pupillary block may occur, and an iridectomy is helpful. If the IOP remains uncontrolled, a trabeculectomy may be required. Some surgeons prefer to perform a trabeculectomy as the initial surgical procedure with the anterior chamber washout in order to obtain immediate IOP control and relief of any pupillary block.

**Hemolytic and ghost cell glaucoma**    Hemolytic and/or ghost cell glaucoma may develop after vitreous hemorrhage. In *hemolytic glaucoma* hemoglobin-laden macrophages block the trabecular outflow channels. Red-tinged cells are seen floating in the anterior chamber, and a reddish brown discoloration of the trabecular meshwork is often present.

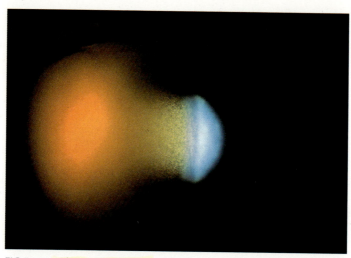

FIG IV-20—Ghost cell glaucoma: the classic appearance of ghost cells in the anterior chamber. These khaki-colored cells are small and can become layered, as is seen in a hyphema and hypopyon. As a result of their loss of pliability, they remain longer in the anterior chamber, causing obstruction of the trabecular meshwork and secondary glaucoma. (Photograph courtesy of Ron Gross, MD.)

Ghost cell glaucoma is a transient secondary open-angle glaucoma caused by degenerated red blood cells (ghost cells) blocking the trabecular meshwork. Ghost cells are red blood cells that have lost their intracellular hemoglobin and appear as small khaki-colored cells that are less pliable than normal red blood cells (Fig IV-20). This loss of pliability results in obstruction of the trabecular meshwork and secondary glaucoma. The cells develop within 1–3 months following a vitreous hemorrhage. They gain access to the anterior chamber through a disrupted hyaloid face, which can occur from previous surgery (pars plana vitrectomy, cataract extraction, or capsulotomy), trauma, or spontaneous disruption.

Clinically, patients present with increased IOP and history of a recent vitreous hemorrhage resulting from trauma, surgery, or preexisting retinal disease. The IOP may be markedly elevated, causing corneal edema. The anterior chamber is filled with small circulating tan-colored cells (see Figure IV-20). The cellular reaction appears out of proportion to the aqueous flare, and the conjunctiva tends not to be inflamed unless the IOP is markedly elevated. Gonioscopically, the angle appears normal except for the layering of ghost cells over the trabecular meshwork inferiorly. The vitreous has the appearance of old hemorrhage with characteristic khaki coloration and clumps of extracellular pigmentation from degenerated hemoglobin.

Both hemolytic and ghost cell glaucoma are generally self-limiting and resolve once the hemorrhage has cleared. Medical therapy with aqueous suppressants is the preferred initial approach. If medical therapy fails to control marked elevations of IOP, some patients may require irrigation of the anterior chamber, pars plana vitrectomy, and/or a trabeculectomy to control the condition.

***Surgical trauma***   Operative procedures such as cataract extraction, filtering surgery, or corneal transplantation may be followed by an increase in IOP. Similarly, laser surgery—including trabeculoplasty, iridectomy, and posterior capsulotomy—may be complicated by posttreatment IOP elevation. Although the IOP may rise as high as 50 mm Hg or more, these elevations are usually transient, lasting from a few hours to a few days. The exact mechanism is not known, but pigment release, presence of inflammatory cells and debris, and mechanical deformation of the trabecular meshwork and angle closure have all been implicated.

In addition, agents used as adjuncts to intraocular surgery may cause secondary IOP elevations. For example, the injection of viscoelastic substances such as sodium hyaluronate into the anterior chamber may result in a transient and possibly severe postoperative increase in IOP. Dispersive viscoelastics (sodium hyaluronate) may be more likely to cause IOP increases than retentive viscoelastic agents (chondroitin sulfate).

Such postoperative pressure elevation can cause considerable damage to the optic nerve of a susceptible individual even in a short time. Eyes with preexisting glaucoma are at particular risk for further damage. Elevated IOP may increase the risk of retinal and optic nerve ischemia. It is thus important to measure IOP soon after surgery or laser treatment. If a substantial rise in IOP does occur, ocular hypertensive therapy may be required. Usually, use of beta-adrenergic antagonists, alpha$_2$-adrenergic agonists, or carbonic anhydrase inhibitors is adequate. However, hyperosmotic agents are sometimes necessary. See chapter VII, Medical Management of Glaucoma, for discussion of these agents.

The implantation of an intraocular lens (IOL) can lead to a variety of secondary glaucomas:

◻ Uveitis-hyphema-glaucoma syndrome (UGH syndrome, Fig IV-21)

◻ Secondary pigmentary glaucoma (Fig IV-22)

◻ Pseudophakic pupillary block (see chapter V)

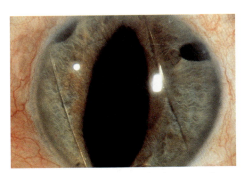

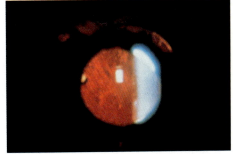

FIG IV-21—Uveitis-glaucoma-hyphema syndrome (UGH) is a form of secondary inflammatory glaucoma caused by chronic inflammation from a malpositioned anterior chamber intraocular lens. The early rigid anterior chamber IOLs, such as this one, were more susceptible to this entity than the more modern lenses used today. (Photograph courtesy of L.J. Katz, MD.)

FIG IV-22—Secondary pigmentary glaucoma. Superior iris transillumination is seen in this photograph caused by the underlying optic and haptic of the posterior chamber IOL. The release of iris pigmentation can lead to trabecular meshwork dysfunction and secondary glaucoma. (Photograph courtesy of Wills Eye Hospital slide collection, 1986.)

*Uveitis-hyphema-glaucoma syndrome* is a form of secondary inflammatory glaucoma caused by chronic irritation that is usually the result of a malpositioned anterior chamber IOL (see Figure IV-21). Characterized by chronic inflammation, secondary iris neovascularization, and recurrent hyphemas, this condition often results in an intractable form of secondary glaucoma following the chafing of the iris by the IOL or erosion of the lens haptics through the iris or ciliary body. This condition may also occur following implantation of a posterior chamber or suture-fixated IOL.

**Glaucoma and penetrating keratoplasty**   Secondary glaucoma is a common complication of penetrating keratoplasty, and it occurs with increased frequency in the aphakic/pseudophakic patient and with repeat grafts. The different mechanisms of the glaucoma are outlined in Table IV-7. Wound distortion of the trabecular meshwork and angle closure are the most common causes of long-standing glaucoma, and attempts to minimize these secondary glaucomas with oversized donor grafts, peripheral iridectomies, and surgical repair of the iris sphincter have been only partially successful. BCSC Section 8, *External Disease and Cornea,* discusses penetrating keratoplasty in detail.

## Drugs and Glaucoma

*Corticosteroid-induced glaucoma* is an open-angle glaucoma caused by prolonged use of topical, periocular, inhaled, or systemic corticosteroids. It mimics primary open-angle glaucoma in its presentation and clinical course. Approximately one third of all patients will demonstrate some responsiveness to corticosteroids, but only a small percentage will have a clinically significant elevation in IOP. The type and potency of the agent, the means and frequency of its administration, and the susceptibility of the patient all affect the duration of time before the IOP rises and the extent of this rise. A high percentage of patients with primary open-angle glaucoma demonstrate this IOP response to topical corticosteroids. Systemic administration of corticosteroids may also raise IOP in some individuals, although less frequently than topical administration. The elevated IOP is a result of an increased resistance to aqueous outflow in the trabecular meshwork.

TABLE IV-7

MECHANISM OF SECONDARY GLAUCOMA FOLLOWING PENETRATING KERATOPLASTY

| OPEN ANGLE | CLOSED ANGLE |
|---|---|
| Inflammatory | Chronic PAS/angle closure |
| Corticosteroid induced | Pupillary block |
| Viscoelastic | In association with corticosteroid use |
| Wound distortion of trabecular meshwork | Fibrous/epithelial ingrowth |
| Fibrous/epithelial ingrowth | Inflammatory |

Corticosteroid-induced glaucoma may develop at any time during long-term corticosteroid administration. IOP thus needs to be monitored regularly in such patients. Some corticosteroid preparations such as fluorometholone, rimexolone (Vexol), or medrysone are less likely to raise IOP than are prednisolone or dexamethasone. However, even weaker corticosteroids or lower concentrations of stronger drugs can raise IOP in susceptible individuals.

A corticosteroid-induced rise in pressure may cause glaucomatous optic nerve damage in some patients. This condition can mimic primary open-angle glaucoma in the adult or infantile glaucoma in the child.

The cause of the elevation in IOP is not always related to the use of a corticosteroid and may be confounded by underlying ocular disease such as anterior uveitis. Following discontinuation of the corticosteroid, the IOP usually decreases; however, unmasked primary open-angle glaucoma or secondary open-angle inflammatory glaucoma may remain.

Patients with excessive levels of endogenous corticosteroids (e.g., Cushing syndrome) can also develop increased IOP. Generally, IOP returns to normal when the corticosteroid-producing tumor or hyperplastic tissue is excised.

*Cycloplegic drugs* can increase IOP in individuals with open angles. Patients with primary open-angle glaucoma are more susceptible.

Epstein DL, Allingham RR, Schuman JS, eds. *Chandler and Grant's Glaucoma*. 4th ed. Baltimore: Williams & Wilkins; 1997.

Shields MB. *Textbook of Glaucoma*. 4th ed. Baltimore: Williams & Wilkins; 1997.

# CHAPTER V

# Angle-Closure Glaucoma

## Mechanisms and Pathophysiology of Angle Closure

Angle closure develops because apposition of the iris to the trabecular meshwork blocks the drainage of aqueous humor. Conceptually, the mechanisms of angle closure fall into two general categories:

□ Mechanisms that *push* the iris forward from behind

□ Mechanisms that *pull* the iris forward into contact with the trabecular meshwork

Some angle-closure glaucomas do not fall clearly into these categories, such as angle closure in aniridia, plateau iris, and Rieger syndrome.

*Pupillary block,* with forward bowing of the iris, is the most frequent cause of angle closure and is the underlying cause of most cases of primary angle-closure glaucoma. The flow of aqueous from the posterior chamber through the pupil is impeded, and this obstruction creates a pressure gradient between the posterior and anterior chambers, causing the peripheral iris to bow forward against the trabecular meshwork (Fig V-1). This sequence is the mechanism for primary pupillary block associated with acute, subacute, and chronic angle-closure glaucoma.

Angle closure may also occur without pupillary block. The lens–iris diaphragm can be pushed or rotated forward by a posterior segment tumor or another space-occupying process or lesion. Examples of this mechanism include

□ Ciliary body swelling, inflammation, or cysts

□ Aqueous misdirection, also known as *malignant,* or *ciliary block,* glaucoma

□ Posterior segment tumors

□ Contracting retrolental tissue

□ Scleral buckling procedures

□ Conditions predisposing to ciliochoroidal effusions (panretinal photocoagulation and nanophthalmos)

In addition, angle closure can occur when the iris is pulled forward by contraction of a membrane or fibrovascular tissue, as with inflammation, neovascularization, or endothelial proliferation closing the anterior chamber angle.

## Primary Angle-Closure Glaucoma

### Pathophysiology

Patients who develop primary angle-closure glaucoma tend to have small anterior segments and a short axial length, predisposing them to increased relative pupillary block. Age also heightens the risk of relative pupillary block, as the lens grows and iridolenticular contact increases. An angle-closure attack is often precipitated by some minor event, such as pupillary dilation. The dilation to midposition relaxes the

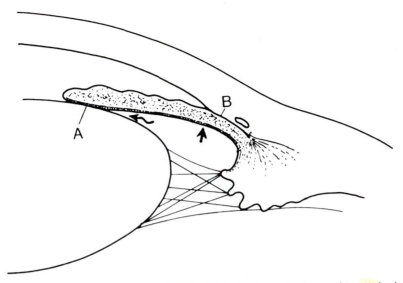

FIG V-1—Pupillary-block glaucoma. A functional block between the lens and iris *(A)* leads to increased pressure in the posterior chamber *(arrows)* with forward shift of the peripheral iris and closure of the anterior chamber angle *(B)*. (Reproduced with permission from Shields MB. *Textbook of Glaucoma.* 3rd ed. Baltimore: Williams & Wilkins; 1992.)

peripheral iris so that it may bow forward, coming into contact with the trabecular meshwork; in this position lens–iris apposition is maximal, setting the stage for pupillary block and subsequent angle closure.

### Acute Primary Angle-Closure Glaucoma

Acute primary angle-closure glaucoma occurs when IOP rises rapidly as a result of relatively sudden blockage of the trabecular meshwork by the iris. It may be manifested by pain, blurred vision, rainbow-colored haloes around lights, nausea, and vomiting. The rise in IOP to relatively high levels causes corneal epithelial edema, which is responsible for the visual symptoms. Signs of acute angle-closure glaucoma include

□ High IOP

□ Middilated, sluggish, and often irregular pupil

□ Corneal epithelial edema

□ Congested episcleral and conjunctival blood vessels

□ Shallow anterior chamber

□ A mild amount of aqueous flare and cells

The optic nerve may be swollen during an acute attack.

Definitive diagnosis depends on the gonioscopic verification of angle closure. Gonioscopy should be possible in almost all cases of acute angle closure, although medical treatment of elevated IOP and clearing of corneal edema with topical glycerin may be necessary to enable visualization of the chamber angle. Compression gonioscopy may help the physician to determine if the iris–trabecular meshwork blockage is reversible (appositional closure) or irreversible (synechial closure), and it may be therapeutic in breaking the attack of acute angle closure. Gonioscopy of the fellow eye in a patient with primary angle-closure glaucoma usually reveals a narrow, occludable angle.

During an acute attack, IOP may be high enough to cause glaucomatous optic nerve damage and/or retinal vascular occlusion. Peripheral anterior synechiae (PAS) can form rapidly, and IOP-induced ischemia may produce sector atrophy of the iris. Such atrophy releases pigment and causes pigmentary dusting of the iris surface and corneal endothelium. Iris ischemia, specifically of the iris sphincter muscle, may cause the pupil to become permanently fixed and dilated. *Glaukomflecken,* characteristic small anterior subcapsular lens opacities, may also develop. These findings are helpful in detecting previous episodes of acute angle-closure glaucoma.

The definitive treatment for acute angle closure is an iridectomy, laser or surgical, which is discussed in detail in chapter VIII. Mild attacks may be broken by cholinergic agents (pilocarpine 1%–2%), which induce miosis that pulls the peripheral iris away from the trabecular meshwork. Stronger miotics should be avoided, as they may increase the vascular congestion of the iris or rotate the lens–iris diaphragm more anteriorly, increasing the pupillary block. However, when the IOP is quite elevated (e.g., above 40–50 mm Hg), the pupillary sphincter may be ischemic and unresponsive to miotic agents alone. The patient should be treated with some combination of a topical beta-adrenergic antagonist; alpha$_2$-adrenergic agonists; an oral, topical, or intravenous carbonic anhydrase inhibitor; and, when necessary, a hyperosmotic agent. This treatment is used to reduce IOP to the point where the miotic agent will constrict the pupil and open the angle. Globe compression and compression gonioscopy have also been described to treat acute angle-closure glaucoma. Nonselective adrenergic agonists or medications with significant alpha$_1$-adrenergic activity (apraclonidine) should be avoided to prevent further pupillary dilation and iris ischemia.

The fellow eye, which shares the anatomic predisposition for increased pupillary block, is at high risk for developing acute angle closure. In addition, the pain and emotional upset resulting from the involvement of the first eye may increase sympathetic flow to the fellow eye and produce pupillary dilation. It is recommended that a peripheral iridectomy be performed in the other eye if a similar angle configuration is present. If it is not, specific secondary angle-closure glaucomas must be strongly considered in the differential diagnosis. In general, primary angle-closure glaucoma is a bilateral disease, and its occurrence in a patient whose fellow eye has a deep chamber angle raises the possibility of a secondary cause, such as a posterior segment mass or iridocorneal endothelial syndrome.

An untreated fellow eye has a 40%–80% chance of developing an acute attack of angle closure over the next 5–10 years. Long-term pilocarpine administration is not effective in preventing acute attacks in many cases, and it may even prevent the detection of chronic angle-closure glaucoma by decreasing the IOP. Thus, prophylactic iridectomy should be performed in the contralateral eye unless the angle clearly appears to be nonoccludable.

Laser iridectomy is the treatment of choice for angle-closure glaucoma secondary to pupillary block. Surgical iridectomy is indicated when laser iridectomy cannot be accomplished. Once an iridectomy has been performed, pupillary block is relieved and the iris is no longer pushed forward into contact with the trabecular meshwork, as the pressure gradient between the posterior and anterior chambers approaches zero. If a laser iridectomy cannot be performed, the acute attack may rarely be stopped by flattening the peripheral iris through iridoplasty or by relieving pupillary block with laser pupilloplasty.

Once the attack is broken, a peripheral iridectomy should be performed as soon as possible. Following resolution of the acute attack, it is important to reevaluate the angle by gonioscopy for persistent residual angle closure that may be amenable to laser gonioplasty. Chapter VIII, Surgical Therapy of Glaucoma, discusses these procedures in detail.

The IOP may remain low for weeks following acute angle-closure glaucoma because of ciliary body ischemia and poor aqueous production, and it is a poor indicator of angle function or anatomy. Repeat or serial gonioscopy is therefore essential.

## Subacute Angle-Closure Glaucoma

Subacute (intermittent or prodromal) angle-closure glaucoma is a condition characterized by episodes of blurred vision, haloes, and mild pain caused by elevated IOP. These symptoms resolve spontaneously, especially during sleep-induced miosis, and IOP is usually normal between the episodes, which occur periodically over days or weeks. These episodes may be confused with headaches or migraines. The correct diagnosis can be made only with a high index of suspicion and gonioscopy. The typical history and the gonioscopic appearance of a narrow chamber angle with or without PAS help establish the diagnosis. Laser iridectomy is the treatment of choice in subacute angle closure. This condition can progress to chronic angle-closure glaucoma or to an acute attack that does not resolve spontaneously.

## Chronic Angle-Closure Glaucoma

This condition may develop either after acute angle closure in which synechial closure persists or when the chamber angle closes gradually and IOP rises slowly as enough angle is compromised. Permanent PAS are present, as determined by indentation gonioscopy. The clinical course resembles that of open-angle glaucoma in its lack of symptoms, modest elevation of IOP, progressive cupping of the optic nerve head, and characteristic glaucomatous loss of visual field. The diagnosis of chronic angle-closure glaucoma is frequently overlooked, and it is commonly confused with chronic open-angle glaucoma. Gonioscopic examination of all glaucoma patients is important to enable the ophthalmologist to make the correct diagnosis.

Even if miotics and other agents lower IOP, iridectomy is necessary to relieve the pupillary block and prevent further permanent synechial angle closure. Without iridectomy, closure of the angle progresses and becomes irreversible. Even with a patent peripheral iridectomy, progressive angle closure infrequently occurs, and repeated periodic gonioscopy is thus imperative. Iridectomy with or without chronic use of ocular hypotensive medication will control the disease for most chronic angle-closure glaucoma patients. Others may require subsequent filtering surgery.

No clinical test can reliably determine whether an iridectomy alone will control the disease for an individual patient. However, since laser iridectomy is a relatively low-risk procedure compared to other surgical procedures, it should be performed prior to a more invasive or risky operative procedure. Individuals with extensive PAS and elevated IOP following acute angle closure may be helped by argon laser gonioplasty or goniosynechialysis.

## The Narrow Anterior Chamber Angle

Only a small percentage of patients with shallow anterior chambers develop angle-closure glaucoma. Many clinicians have attempted to predict which asymptomatic patients with normal IOP will develop angle closure by performing a variety of provocative tests. These tests are designed to precipitate a limited form of angle closure, which can then be detected by gonioscopy and IOP measurement. The methods commonly used include pharmacologic pupillary dilation and prone-darkroom testing. An IOP increase of 8 mm Hg or more is considered positive. An asymmetric pressure rise between the two eyes with a corresponding degree of angle closure is also considered a positive sign. None of the provocative tests has been validated in a prospective study, however, and the predictive value of any provocative test has never been demonstrated. Thus, they are rarely used.

Ultimately, the decision to treat an asymptomatic patient with narrow angles rests on the clinical judgment of the ophthalmologist and the accurate assessment of the anterior chamber angle. Any patient with narrow angles, regardless of the results of provocative testing, should be advised of the symptoms of angle closure, of the need for immediate ophthalmic attention if symptoms occur, and of the value of long-term periodic follow-up. An iridectomy is not necessary in all patients with a suspicious or borderline narrow angle.

Various factors that cause pupillary dilation may induce angle-closure glaucoma. These factors include a variety of drugs as well as pain, emotional upset, or fright. In predisposed eyes with shallow anterior chambers, either mydriatic or miotic agents can precipitate acute angle closure. Mydriatic agents include not only dilating drops but also systemic medications that cause dilation. The effect of miotics is to pull the peripheral iris away from the chamber angle. However, miotics also cause the zonular fibers of the lens to relax, allowing the lens to come forward. Furthermore, their use results in an increase in the amount of iris–lens contact, thus potentially increasing pupillary block. For these reasons, miotics, especially the cholinesterase inhibitors, may also induce or aggravate angle-closure glaucoma. Gonioscopy should be repeated soon after miotic drugs are administered to patients with narrow angles.

A number of systemic medications, including some nonprescription preparations, carry warnings against use by patients with glaucoma. Most of these drugs have the potential for precipitating angle closure in susceptible individuals because of anticholinergic or sympathomimetic activity. While systemic administration generally does not raise intraocular drug levels to the same degree as does topical administration, even slight mydriasis in a patient with a critically narrow chamber angle can induce angle-closure glaucoma. Patients with narrow angles who have not had an iridectomy should be warned about this possibility.

The use of an alpha-adrenergic antagonist has been suggested to reverse the effects of sympathomimetic dilating agents and minimize the chances of angle closure. Moxisylyte (thymoxamine), which is not commercially available, and dapiprazole, available in a 0.5% solution, both reverse phenylephrine- or tropicamide-induced pupillary dilation to baseline in 30 minutes compared with 3 hours when no alpha-adrenergic antagonist is used. However, this suggested combination of alpha-adrenergic agonist and adrenergic antagonist does not eliminate the possibility of precipitating angle closure; it just allows the pupil to constrict through the critical middilation stage more quickly. Moxisylyte has also been used as a diagnostic test for combined-mechanism glaucoma. Because it produces miosis without affecting the ciliary body–controlled facility of outflow, it can sometimes open a narrow or appositionally closed angle and separate the angle-closure component from the open-angle component in combined-mechanism glaucoma.

## Plateau Iris

Plateau iris is an unusual type of primary angle-closure glaucoma caused by anteriorly positioned ciliary processes that critically narrow the anterior chamber recess by pushing the peripheral iris forward. A component of pupillary block is often present. Following dilation of the pupil, the peripheral iris bunches up and obstructs the trabecular meshwork. Plateau iris may be suspected if the central anterior chamber seems unusually deep and the iris plane appears rather flat for an eye with angle closure. This suspicion can be confirmed with ultrasound biomicroscopy (Fig V-2). The

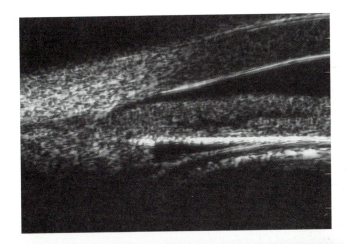

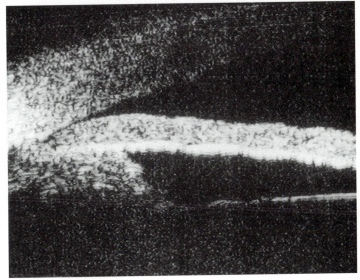

FIG V-2—Ultrasound biomicroscopy images of a plateau iris. (Photographs courtesy of Charles J. Pavlin, MD.)

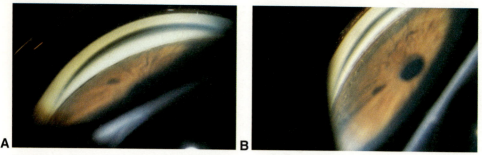

FIG V-3—*A*, Plateau iris syndrome with a flat iris plane and closed angle. *B*, Plateau iris syndrome with an open angle following laser peripheral iridoplasty.

ophthalmologist should also suspect plateau iris if angle closure occurs in younger myopic patients.

An iridectomy is performed to remove any component of pupillary block; this treatment is sufficient for eyes with *plateau iris configuration,* the more common manifestation. However, even after iridectomy, a few eyes with *plateau iris syndrome* will still be predisposed to develop angle closure as a result of the peripheral iris anatomy. These patients should be treated with long-term miotic therapy. Laser peripheral iridoplasty to thin the peripheral iris is often useful in individuals with this condition to flatten the peripheral iris (Fig V-3). Repeat gonioscopy is necessary, as the peripheral iris may bow anteriorly again over time.

## Secondary Angle-Closure Glaucoma with Pupillary Block

### Lens-Induced Angle-Closure Glaucoma

Intumescent or dislocated lenses (complete zonular dehiscence) may increase pupillary block and cause angle-closure glaucoma. Angle closure from a swollen lens is sometimes referred to as *phacomorphic glaucoma.* With lens subluxation (partial zonular dehiscence), as in Marfan syndrome or homocystinuria, pupillary block from the lens or vitreous may occur. See also BCSC Section 11, *Lens and Cataract.*

***Phacomorphic glaucoma*** As with primary angle closure, lens size and relative pupillary block play vital roles in this condition. The main difference is that primary angle closure tends to occur slowly in hyperopes who undergo progressive shallowing of the anterior chamber as a result of increasing anterior–posterior lens diameter. The process in phacomorphic glaucoma is much more rapid and is precipitated by marked lens swelling (intumescence) as a result of cataract formation and the development of pupillary block in an eye anatomically not disposed to closure (Figs V-4, V-5). As a result of the similarities, diagnosis is not always straightforward, but disparities between the two eyes in the anterior chamber depths and degree of cataract should suggest a phacomorphic process (Fig V-6).

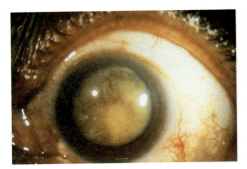

FIG V-4—Phacomorphic glaucoma. Lens intumescence precipitates pupillary block and secondary angle closure in an eye not anatomically predisposed to angle closure.

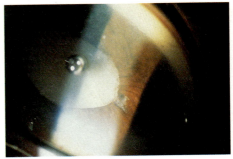

FIG V-5—Phacomorphic glaucoma. Classic iris bombé develops as a result of a mature cataract and secondary posterior synechiae.

***Ectopia lentis*** Ectopia lentis is defined as displacement of the lens from its normal anatomic position. Anterior displacement of the lens can result in pupillary block by itself or in combination with the vitreous (Fig V-7). The pupillary block causes iris bombé and shallowing of the anterior chamber angle to occur, with resultant secondary angle-closure glaucoma. This may present clinically as an acute event with pain, conjunctival hyperemia, and loss of vision or as a chronic angle-closure glaucoma with PAS formation secondary to repeated attacks. Laser iridectomy is the treatment of choice, as it is with primary angle-closure glaucoma with pupillary block. Lens extraction is indicated if pupillary block is not relieved or when the ante-

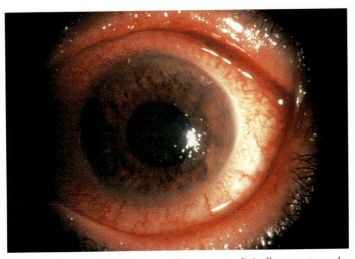

FIG V-6—Phacomorphic glaucoma often presents clinically as acute angle-closure glaucoma. Disparities in the anterior chamber depths and degree of cataract between the two eyes can help the clinician distinguish between a phacomorphic process and primary angle-closure glaucoma.

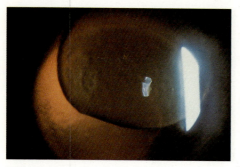

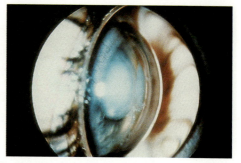

FIG V-7—Ectopia lentis: dislocation of the lens into the anterior chamber through a dilated pupil. (Photograph courtesy of Ron Gross, MD.)

FIG V-8—Ectopia lentis. In a case of microspherophakia, the lens is trapped anteriorly by the pupil, resulting in iris bombé and a dramatic shallowing of the anterior chamber. (Photograph courtesy of G.L. Spaeth, MD.)

rior chamber progressively shallows following laser iridectomy. A list of conditions causing this entity is given in Table V-1.

*Microspherophakia,* a congenital disorder in which the lens has a spherical or globular shape, may cause pupillary block and angle-closure glaucoma (Fig V-8). Treatment with cycloplegia may flatten the lens and pull it posteriorly, breaking the pupillary block. Miotics may make the glaucoma worse. Microspherophakia is often familial and may occur as an isolated condition or as part of either Weill-Marchesani or Marfan syndrome.

**Aphakic or pseudophakic angle-closure glaucoma**   Pupillary block may occur in *aphakic* and *pseudophakic* eyes. An intact vitreous face can block the pupil and/or an iridectomy in aphakic or pseudophakic eyes or in phakic eyes with dislocated lenses. Generally, the anterior chamber shallows and the iris demonstrates considerable bombé. Treatment with mydriatic and cycloplegic agents may restore the

TABLE V-1

COMMON CAUSES OF ECTOPIA LENTIS

Trauma

Marfan syndrome

Homocystinuria

Microspherophakia

Weill-Marchesani syndrome

aqueous flow through the pupil but may also make the performing of a laser iridectomy difficult initially. Topical beta-adrenergic antagonists, alpha$_2$-adrenergic agonists, carbonic anhydrase inhibitors, and hyperosmotic agents can be effective in reducing the IOP prior to the placement of an iridectomy. One or more laser iridectomies may be required.

A variant of this problem occurs with *anterior chamber intraocular lenses*. Pupillary block develops with apposition of the iris, vitreous face, and/or lens optic. The lens haptic or vitreous may obstruct the iridectomy or the pupil, and the peripheral iris bows forward around the anterior chamber IOL to occlude the chamber angle. The central chamber remains deep in this instance, because the lens haptic and optic prevent the central portions of the iris and vitreous face from moving forward. Laser iridectomies, often multiple, are required to relieve the block.

Pupillary block may occur after *extracapsular cataract extraction* when an iridectomy has not been performed at the time of surgery. Although not common, this complication can occur when the iris forms adhesions to a posterior chamber IOL or to the residual anterior or posterior capsule. Pupillary block may also occur following posterior capsulotomy when vitreous obstructs the pupil. A condition referred to as capsular block may also be seen whereby retained viscoelastic or fluid in the capsular bag pushes a posterior chamber IOL anteriorly, which may narrow the angle.

### Nonrhegmatogenous Retinal Detachment

Subretinal effusion where no retinal breaks are present may cause nonrhegmatogenous retinal detachment. Retinoblastoma, Coats disease, metastatic carcinoma, choroidal melanoma, and subretinal neovascularization in age-related macular degeneration with extensive effusion or hemorrhage are associated with this condition. See BCSC Section 12, *Retina and Vitreous*, for further discussion.

In a *rhegmatogenous retinal detachment* the subretinal fluid can escape through the retinal tear and equalize the hydraulic pressure on both sides of the retina. In a nonrhegmatogenous retinal detachment, by contrast, the subretinal fluid accumulates and progressively pushes the retina forward against the lens like a hydraulic press. The fluid or hemorrhage may accumulate rapidly, and as it pushes the bullous retinal detachment forward to a retrolenticular position, it can flatten the anterior chamber completely. The retina may be dramatically visible behind the lens on slit-lamp examination. The creation of a retinotomy, like an iridectomy in acute angle-closure glaucoma, relieves the increased IOP by equalizing the hydraulic pressure in front of and behind the retina and allows the retina to fall posteriorly.

## Secondary Angle-Closure Glaucoma without Pupillary Block

A number of disorders can lead to secondary angle-closure glaucoma without pupillary block, and several are discussed in this section. This form of secondary angle closure may occur through one of two mechanisms:

□ Contraction of a membrane, band, or exudate in the angle, leading to peripheral anterior synechiae

□ Forward displacement of the lens–iris diaphragm, often accompanied by swelling and anterior rotation of the ciliary body

TABLE V-2

DISORDERS PREDISPOSING TO NEOVASCULARIZATION OF THE IRIS AND ANGLE

**Systemic vascular disease**
Carotid occlusive disease*
Carotid artery ligation
Carotid cavernous fistula
Giant cell arteritis
Takayasu (pulseless) disease

**Ocular vascular disease**
Diabetic retinopathy*
Central retinal vein occlusion*
Central retinal artery occlusion
Branch retinal vein occlusion
Sickle cell retinopathy
Coats disease
Eales disease
Retinopathy of prematurity
Persistent hyperplastic primary vitreous
Syphilitic vasculitis
Anterior segment ischemia

**Other ocular disease**
Chronic uveitis
Chronic retinal detachment
Endophthalmitis
Stickler syndrome
Retinoschisis

**Intraocular tumors**
Uveal melanoma
Metastatic carcinoma
Retinoblastoma
Reticulum cell sarcoma

**Ocular therapy**
Radiation therapy

**Trauma**

*most common causes

## Neovascular Glaucoma

This common, severe type of secondary angle-closure glaucoma is caused by a variety of disorders characterized by retinal or ocular ischemia or ocular inflammation (Table V-2). The disease is characterized by fine arborizing blood vessels on the surface of the iris and trabecular meshwork, which are accompanied by a fibrous membrane. The contraction of the fibrovascular membrane results in the formation of PAS, leading to the development of secondary angle-closure glaucoma.

Neovascularization of the anterior segment usually presents in a classic pattern that starts with fine vascular tufts at the pupil (Fig V-9). As these vessels grow, they extend radially over the iris. The neovascularization crosses the ciliary body and scleral spur as fine single vessels that then branch as they reach and involve the trabecular meshwork (Figs V-10, V-11). Often the trabecular meshwork takes on a reddish coloration. With contraction of the fibrovascular membrane, PAS develop and coalesce, gradually closing the angle (Fig V-12). Because the fibrovascular membrane cannot grow over healthy corneal endothelium, the PAS end at Schwalbe's line, distinguishing this condition from other secondary angle-closure glaucomas that result from an abnormal corneal endothelium such as ICE syndrome, which is discussed below (Figs V-13, V-14).

Clinically, patients often present with an acute glaucoma associated with reduced vision, pain, conjunctival injection, microcystic corneal edema, and high IOP. If excessive pressure is applied during gonioscopy, fine neovascularization can be blanched, confusing this condition with acute angle closure, especially if corneal edema is present.

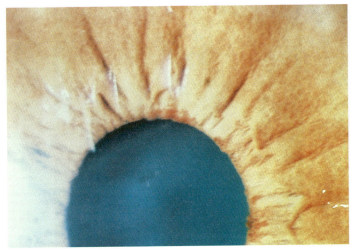

FIG V-9—The initial presentation of iris neovascularization is usually small vascular tufts at the pupillary margin.

Rarely, anterior segment neovascularization may occur without demonstrable retinal ischemia, as in Fuchs heterochromic iridocyclitis and other types of uveitis, exfoliation syndrome, or isolated iris melanomas. When an ocular cause cannot be found, carotid artery occlusive disease should be considered. In establishing a correct diagnosis, it is important to distinguish dilated iris vessels associated with inflammation from newly formed abnormal blood vessels.

Because the prognosis for neovascular glaucoma is poor, prevention is desirable. The most common cause of iris neovascularization is ischemic retinopathy, and

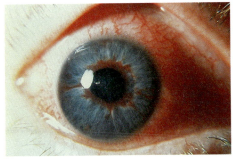

FIG V-10—With growth, iris neovascularization extends from the pupillary margin radially toward the anterior chamber angle.

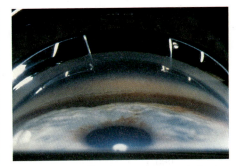

FIG V-11—Initially, the iris neovascularization crosses the angle recess and scleral spur as single vessels that then branch over the trabecular meshwork. (Photograph courtesy of Tom Richardson, MD.)

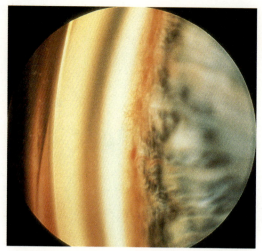

FIG V-12—Iris neovascularization. With progressive angle involvement, peripheral anterior synechiae develop with contraction of the fibrovascular membrane, resulting in secondary neovascular glaucoma.

retinal ablation should be performed whenever possible. The treatment of choice when the ocular media are clear is panretinal photocoagulation. When cloudy media prevent laser therapy, panretinal cryotherapy should be considered versus surgery to clear the media with associated panretinal photocoagulation. Frequently, marked involution of the neovascularization occurs. The resulting decrease in neovascularization after retinal ablation may reduce or normalize the IOP, depending on

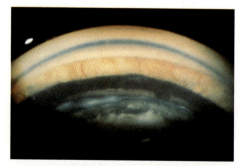

FIG V-13—With endstage neovascular glaucoma, total angle closure occurs, obscuring the iris neovascularization. The PAS end at Schwalbe's line because the fibrovascular membrane does not grow over healthy corneal endothelium.

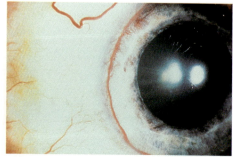

FIG V-14—Often a large single vessel outlines the end of the PAS at the level of Schwalbe's line.

the degree of synechial closure that has occurred. Even in the presence of total synechial angle closure, panretinal photocoagulation may improve the success rate of filtering surgery by eliminating the angiogenic stimulus and decrease the risk of hemorrhage at the time of surgery.

Medical therapy is usually not effective in controlling IOP when the outflow system has been occluded. However, topical beta-adrenergic antagonists, alpha$_2$-adrenergic agonists, carbonic anhydrase inhibitors, cycloplegics, and corticosteroids may be useful in reducing IOP and decreasing inflammation. Filtering surgery has a better chance of success once neovascularization has regressed after panretinal photocoagulation. The use of the antimetabolites 5-fluorouracil and mitomycin-C has been shown to increase the success rate and decrease the final IOP following filtering surgery in this population. A variety of tube-shunt operations can also be effective in controlling the IOP in neovascular glaucoma, but if these fail, a cyclodestructive procedure may help reduce IOP.

## Iridocorneal Endothelial (ICE) Syndrome

Iridocorneal endothelial syndrome is a group of disorders characterized by abnormal corneal endothelium that causes variable degrees of iris atrophy, secondary angle-closure glaucoma, and corneal edema. BCSC Section 8, *External Disease and Cornea,* discusses the corneal aspects of ICE syndrome. Three clinical variants have been described:

□ Chandler syndrome

□ Progressive iris atrophy

□ Cogan-Reese syndrome

The condition is clinically unilateral, presents between 20 and 50 years of age, and occurs more often in women. Patients present complaining of decreased vision, pain secondary to corneal edema or secondary angle-closure glaucoma, or an abnormal iris appearance. In each of the three clinical variants the corneal endothelium appears abnormal and takes on a beaten bronze appearance, similar to corneal guttatae seen in Fuchs corneal endothelial dystrophy (Fig V-15). Microcystic corneal edema may be present without elevated IOP, especially in Chandler syndrome. The unaffected eye may have subtle changes of the corneal endothelium without other manifestations of the disease.

High peripheral anterior synechiae are characteristic of ICE syndrome, and these often extend anterior to Schwalbe's line (Fig V-16). The PAS are caused by the contraction of the single layer of endothelial cells and surrounding collagenous-fibrillar tissue that extend from the peripheral cornea over the trabecular meshwork and iris. These PAS result in synechial closure of the anterior chamber angle and lead to an angle-closure glaucoma. Similar to neovascular glaucoma, the degree of angle closure does not always correlate to the elevation in IOP, since some angles may be functionally closed by the endothelial membrane without synechial formation.

Various degrees of iris atrophy and corneal changes distinguish the specific clinical entities. Progressive iris atrophy is characterized by severe iris atrophy resulting in heterochromia, corectopia, ectropion uveae, iris stromal and pigment epithelial atrophy, and hole formation (Fig V-17). In Chandler syndrome minimal iris atrophy and corectopia occurs and the corneal and angle findings predominate (Figs V-18, V-19). Similarly, the iris atrophy tends to be less severe in Cogan-Reese syndrome.

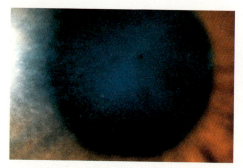

FIG V-15—In all clinical varieties of iridocorneal endothelial syndrome, the corneal endothelium appears abnormal and takes on the appearance of hammered silver, as demonstrated in this patient with Chandler syndrome.

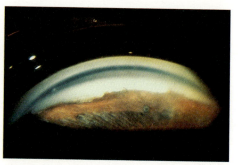

FIG V-16—The classic high peripheral anterior synechiae seen in iridocorneal endothelial syndrome. These PAS extend anterior to Schwalbe's line in this patient with progressive iris atrophy. With angle closure, the secondary glaucoma occurs.

This condition is distinguished by tan pedunculated nodules or diffuse pigmented lesions on the anterior iris surface.

A viral cause has been postulated for the mechanism of ICE syndrome after lymphocytes were seen on the corneal endothelium of affected patients. Both Epstein-Barr and herpes simplex viruses have been implicated in serological studies.

The diagnosis of ICE syndrome must always be considered in young to middle-aged patients who present with unilateral angle-closure glaucoma. Specular microscopy can confirm the diagnosis. Therapy is directed toward the corneal edema

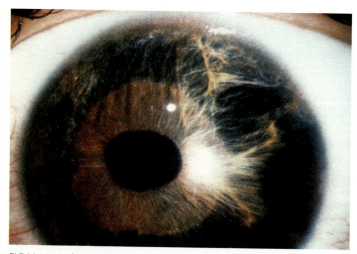

FIG V-17—Iridocorneal endothelial syndrome. Corectopia and hole formation are typical findings in progressive iris atrophy.

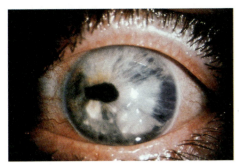 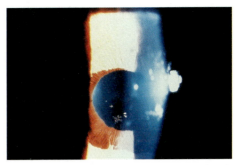

FIG V-18—Iridocorneal endothelial syndrome. The iris atrophy is less severe in Chandler syndrome, but corectopia and bullous keratopathy are seen in this patient.

FIG V-19—Ectropion uveae in a patient with Chandler syndrome.

and secondary glaucoma. Hypertonic saline solutions and medications to reduce the IOP, when elevated, can be effective in controlling the corneal edema. The angle-closure glaucoma can be treated medically with aqueous suppressants. Miotics are ineffective, and the role of prostaglandin analogues remains uncertain. When medical therapy fails, filtering surgery (trabeculectomy or tube-shunt procedures) can be effective. Late failures have been reported with trabeculectomy secondary to fistular endothelialization. These can be reopened in some cases with an Nd:YAG laser.

## Tumors

Tumors in the posterior segment of the eye or anterior uveal cysts may force the lens–iris diaphragm forward and cause angle-closure glaucoma. Uveal melanomas are the most common type of tumors causing angle-closure glaucoma. Extensive tumors of the posterior pole may also cause neovascular glaucoma.

## Inflammation

Secondary angle-closure glaucoma can result from ocular inflammation. Fibrin and increased aqueous proteins from the breakdown of the blood–aqueous barrier predispose the eye to the formation of posterior synechiae (Fig V-20). If left untreated, these synechiae can result in iris bombé and secondary angle closure (Fig V-21).

Inflammation may prompt PAS to form through peripheral iris edema, organization of inflammatory debris in the angle, and the bridging of the angle by large KP. Unlike primary angle closure, where the PAS occur preferentially in the superior angle, they occur most frequently in inflammatory disease in the inferior angle (Fig V-22). These PAS tend to be nonuniform in shape and height, which further differentiates inflammatory disease from primary angle closure (Fig V-23). Ischemia secondary to inflammation may rarely cause rubeosis iridis and neovascular glaucoma.

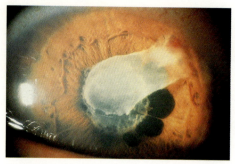

FIG V-20—Inflammatory glaucoma. A fibrinous anterior chamber reaction and posterior synechiae formation are shown in a patient with ankylosing spondylitis.

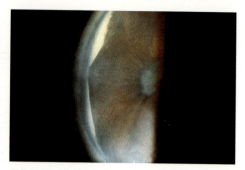

FIG V-21—Inflammatory glaucoma. A secluded pupil is shown in a patient with long-standing uveitis with classic iris bombé and secondary angle closure.

Ocular inflammation can lead to the shallowing and closure of the anterior chamber angle by uveal effusion, resulting in anterior rotation of the ciliary body. Significant posterior uveitis causing massive exudative retinal detachment may lead to angle-closure glaucoma through forward displacement of the lens–iris diaphragm. Treatment is primarily directed at the underlying cause of uveitis. Aqueous suppressants and corticosteroids are the primary agents for reducing elevated IOP and preventing synechial angle closure.

Interstitial keratitis may be associated with open-angle or angle-closure glaucoma. The angle closure may be caused by chronic inflammation and PAS formation or by multiple cysts of the iris pigment epithelium.

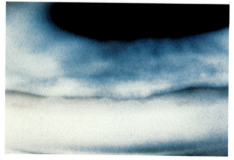

FIG V-22—Inflammatory glaucoma. Keratic precipitates can be seen bridging the inferior anterior chamber angle in this patient with long-standing uveitis, resulting in the formation of PAS. (Photograph courtesy of Joseph Krug, MD.)

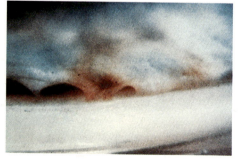

FIG V-23—Inflammatory glaucoma. PAS in uveitis occur preferentially in the inferior anterior chamber angle and are nonuniform in height and shape, as demonstrated in this photograph. (Photograph courtesy of Joseph Krug, MD.)

## Aqueous Misdirection

Aqueous misdirection is also known as *malignant glaucoma, ciliary block glaucoma,* and *posterior aqueous diversion syndrome.* This rare but potentially devastating form of glaucoma usually presents following ocular surgery in patients with a history of angle closure or PAS. It may also occur spontaneously in eyes with an open angle following cataract surgery or various laser procedures. The disease presents with uniform flattening of the anterior chamber, in contrast to iris bombé, and an elevated IOP, usually following incisional surgery. The condition is thought to result from anterior rotation of the ciliary body and posterior misdirection of the aqueous in association with a relative block to aqueous movement at the level of the lens equator, vitreous face, and ciliary processes.

Clinically, the anterior chamber is shallow or flat with anterior displacement of the lens, pseudophakos, or vitreous face. Ciliary processes are seen to be rotated anteriorly and may be seen through an iridectomy to come in contact with the lens equator. Optically clear "aqueous" zones may be seen in the vitreous highlighting the underlying pathology. In the early postoperative setting, the diagnosis of aqueous misdirection is often difficult to distinguish from a choroidal effusion, pupillary block, or a suprachoroidal hemorrhage. Often the level of IOP, time frame following surgery, patency of an iridectomy, or presence of a choroidal effusion or suprachoroidal hemorrhage help the clinician make the appropriate diagnosis and initiate treatment. In some cases, unfortunately, the clinical picture is difficult to interpret and surgical intervention may be required to make the diagnosis.

*[handwritten margin note: pupillary block(?) & en quienes no se extrajo el cristalino]*

Medical management includes intensive cycloplegic therapy, beta-adrenergic antagonists, alpha$_2$-adrenergic agonists, carbonic anhydrase inhibitors, and hyperosmotic agents. Miotics should not be used and can make aqueous misdirection worse. Prostaglandin analogues have not been evaluated but would appear to be contraindicated, as they may increase inflammation. In aphakic and pseudophakic eyes, the anterior vitreous can be disrupted with the Nd:YAG laser. Argon laser photocoagulation of the ciliary processes has reportedly been helpful in treating this condition; this procedure may alter the adjacent vitreous face. The surgical treatment is a vitrectomy combined with anterior chamber deepening. BCSC Section 12, *Retina and Vitreous,* discusses vitrectomy in greater detail.

Lundy DC. Ciliary block glaucoma. In: *Focal Points: Clinical Modules for Ophthalmologists.* San Francisco: American Academy of Ophthalmology; 1999: vol 17, no 3.

*[handwritten note: GLAUCOMA MALIGNO = CILIARY BLOCK GLAUCOMA = POSTERIOR AQUEOUS DIVERSION SYNDROME]*

## Downgrowth

...liferation are rare surgical complications that can cause ...ucomas. Fortunately, improved surgical and wound clo...ly reduced the incidence of these entities (Fig V-24). ...n can be present in three forms: "pearl" tumors of the ...pithelial ingrowth. The latter two often cause secondary ...appear as translucent, nonvascular anterior chamber cysts that originate from the surgical or traumatic wound (Fig V-25). Epithelial ingrowth presents as a grayish sheetlike growth on the trabecular meshwork, iris, ciliary body, and posterior surface of the cornea. It is often associated with wound incarceration, wound gape, ocular inflammation, and corneal edema (Figs V-26, V-27).

The argon laser produces characteristic white burns on the epithelial membrane on the iris surface, which helps to confirm the diagnosis of epithelial downgrowth

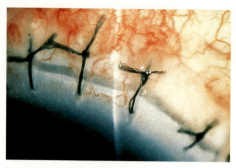

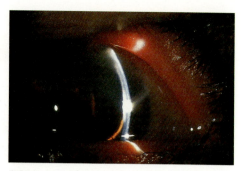

FIG V-24—Epithelial and fibrous proliferation. This corneal scleral wound gape occurred following cataract extraction with silk closure of the incision. Improved surgical and wound closure techniques have greatly reduced the incidence of epithelial and fibrous proliferation. (Photograph courtesy of Wills Eye Hospital slide collection, 1986.)

FIG V-25—Epithelial cysts appear as translucent, nonvascular anterior chamber cysts that originate from a surgical or traumatic wound. The two large cysts shown in this photograph originated from a cataract incision.

and to determine the extent of involvement. If the diagnosis remains in question, a cytologic examination of an aqueous aspirate can be performed. Radical surgery is recommended to remove the intraocular epithelial membrane and the affected tissues and to repair the fistula, but the prognosis remains poor.

Fibrovascular tissue may also proliferate into an eye from a penetrating wound. Unlike epithelial proliferation, fibrous ingrowth progresses slowly and is often self-limited. A common cause of corneal graft failure, fibrous ingrowth appears as a thick, gray-white, vascular, retrocorneal membrane with an irregular border. The

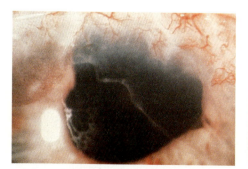

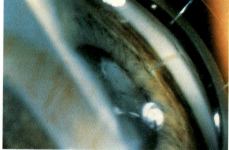

FIG V-26—Epithelial ingrowth appears as a grayish sheetlike growth on the endothelial surface of the cornea, usually originating from a surgical incision or traumatic wound. The epithelial ingrowth shown here originates from a cataract incision.

FIG V-27—Epithelial ingrowth. The precipitating causes of epithelial ingrowth include vitreous incarceration in corneal and scleral wounds, as seen in this photograph, as well as wound gape, ocular inflammation, and hypotony secondary to choroidal effusions.

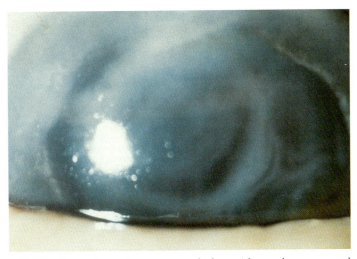

FIG V-28—Fibrous ingrowth appears as a thick, grayish vascular retrocorneal membrane that results in high peripheral anterior synechiae and destruction of the trabecular meshwork.

ingrowth often involves the angle, resulting in PAS and the destruction of the trabecular meshwork (Fig V-28). The resultant secondary angle-closure glaucoma is often difficult to control. Medication is the preferred treatment of the secondary glaucoma, although surgical intervention may be required. See chapter VII, Medical Management of Glaucoma, and chapter VIII, Surgical Therapy of Glaucoma, for detailed discussion.

### Trauma

Angle-closure glaucoma without pupillary block may develop following ocular trauma from the formation of PAS associated with angle recession or from contusion, hyphema, and inflammation. See chapter IV for discussion of trauma.

### Retinal Surgery and Retinal Vascular Disease

Angle-closure glaucoma may occur following treatment of retinal disorders, and it is important to measure IOP after retinal detachment surgery. Scleral buckling operations, especially encircling bands, can produce shallowing of the anterior chamber angle and frank angle-closure glaucoma, often accompanied by choroidal effusion and anterior rotation of the ciliary body, causing a flattening of the peripheral iris with a relatively deep central anterior chamber. Usually, the anterior chamber deepens with the opening of the anterior chamber angle over days to weeks with therapy of cycloplegics, anti-inflammatory agents, beta-adrenergic antagonists, carbonic anhydrase inhibitors, and hyperosmotic agents. If medical management is unsuccessful, argon laser gonioplasty, drainage of suprachoroidal fluid, or adjustment of the scleral buckle is required. Iridectomy is usually of little benefit in this condition.

The scleral buckle can impede venous drainage by compressing a vortex vein, increasing episcleral venous pressure and IOP. Only by shifting the scleral buckle or releasing the band can this elevation in IOP be treated permanently.

Following pars plana vitreous surgery, angle-closure glaucoma may result from the injection of air, long-acting gases such as sulfur hexafluoride and perfluorocarbons (perfluoropropane and perfluoroethane), or silicone oil. These substances are less dense than water and rise to the top of the eye, and an iridectomy may be beneficial. The iridectomy should be located inferiorly to prevent obstruction of the iridectomy site by the oil or gas. Eyes that have undergone complicated vitreoretinal surgery and have developed elevated IOP require individualized treatment plans. Treatment options include the following:

□ Removal of silicone oil

□ Releasing of the encircling element

□ Removal of expansile gases

□ Filtering surgery including tube-shunts

□ Cilioablation

Following panretinal photocoagulation, IOP may become elevated by an angle-closure mechanism. The ciliary body is thickened and rotated, and often an anterior annular choroidal detachment occurs. Generally, this secondary glaucoma is self-limited, and therapy is directed at temporary medical management with cycloplegic agents, topical corticosteroids, and aqueous suppressants.

Central retinal vein occlusion (CRVO) sometimes causes early shallowing of the chamber angle, presumably because of swelling of the choroid and ciliary body. In rare cases the angle becomes sufficiently compromised to cause angle-closure glaucoma. The chamber deepens and the glaucoma resolves over 1 to several weeks. Medical therapy of the glaucoma is usually preferred in combination with topical corticosteroids and cycloplegia. However, if the contralateral eye of a patient with CRVO has a potentially occludable anterior chamber angle, the ophthalmologist must consider an underlying pupillary-block mechanism and the possible need for bilateral iridectomy.

## Nanophthalmos

A nanophthalmic eye is normal in shape but unusually small, with a shortened anteroposterior diameter, a small corneal diameter, and a relatively large lens for the eye volume. Thickened sclera may impede drainage from the vortex veins. These eyes are markedly hyperopic and highly susceptible to primary angle-closure glaucoma. Intraocular surgery is frequently complicated by choroidal effusion and non-rhegmatogenous retinal detachment. Choroidal effusion may occur spontaneously, and it can induce angle-closure glaucoma. Laser iridectomy, argon laser peripheral iridoplasty, and medical therapy are the safest ways to manage glaucoma in these patients.

## Fuchs Corneal Endothelial Dystrophy

Eyes with Fuchs corneal endothelial dystrophy and shallow anterior chamber angles may develop angle-closure glaucoma caused by a gradual thickening of the cornea from edema, resulting in eventual closure of the anterior chamber angle. See BCSC Section 8, *External Disease and Cornea*, for further discussion.

## Retinopathy of Prematurity

Contracting retrolental tissue seen in retinopathy of prematurity (retrolental fibropla-sia) and persistent hyperplastic primary vitreous (PHPV) can cause progressive shal-lowing of the anterior chamber angle with subsequent angle-closure glaucoma. These conditions are discussed in more detail in BCSC Section 6, *Pediatric Oph-thalmology and Strabismus,* and Section 12, *Retina and Vitreous.* In retinopathy of prematurity the onset of this complication usually occurs at 3–6 months of age dur-ing the cicatricial phase of the disease. However, the angle-closure glaucoma may occur later in childhood.

PHPV is usually unilateral and often associated with microphthalmos and elon-gated ciliary processes. The contracture of the hyperplastic primary vitreous and swelling of a cataractous lens may result in subsequent angle-closure glaucoma.

## Flat Anterior Chamber

A flat anterior chamber from any cause can result in the formation of PAS. Debate continues concerning how long a postoperative flat chamber should be treated con-servatively before surgical intervention is undertaken. Hypotony in an eye with a postoperative flat chamber following cataract surgery often indicates a wound leak, and a Seidel test should be performed to locate the leak. Simple pressure patching or bandage contact lens application will often cause the leak to seal and the cham-ber to re-form. If the chamber does not re-form, it should be repaired surgically to prevent permanent synechial closure of the angle.

Some ophthalmologists repair the wound leak and re-form a flat chamber fol-lowing cataract surgery within 24 hours. Others prefer corticosteroid therapy for several days to prevent synechiae formation. If the hyaloid face or an IOL is in con-tact with the cornea, the chambers should be re-formed without delay to mini-mize corneal endothelial damage. Early intervention should also be considered in the presence of corneal edema, excessive inflammation, or posterior synechiae formation.

Epstein DL, Allingham RR, Schuman JS, eds. *Chandler and Grant's Glaucoma.* 4th ed. Baltimore: Williams & Wilkins; 1997.

Ritch R, Shields MB, Krupin T, eds. *The Glaucomas.* 2nd ed. St Louis: Mosby; 1996.

Shields MB. *Textbook of Glaucoma.* 4th ed. Baltimore: Williams & Wilkins; 1997.

Stamper RL, Lieberman MF, Drake MV, eds. *Becker-Shaffer's Diagnosis and Therapy of the Glaucomas.* 7th ed. St Louis: Mosby; 1999.

# CHAPTER VI

# Childhood Glaucoma

BCSC Section 6, *Pediatric Ophthalmology and Strabismus,* also discusses the issues covered here in chapter XXI, Pediatric Glaucomas.

## Definitions and Classification

*Primary congenital* or *infantile glaucoma* is evident either at birth or within the first few years of life. Both conditions are believed to be caused by dysplasia of the anterior chamber angle without other ocular or systemic abnormalities. *Secondary infantile glaucoma* is associated with inflammatory, neoplastic, hamartomatous, metabolic, or other congenital abnormalities of the eye. *Juvenile glaucoma* is recognized later in childhood (after 3 years of age) or in early adulthood.

The term *developmental glaucoma* includes primary congenital glaucoma and glaucoma associated with other developmental anomalies, either ocular or systemic. Glaucoma associated with other ocular or systemic abnormalities may be inherited or acquired. The term *buphthalmos* (cow's eye) refers to enlargement of the globe. This condition appears when the onset of elevated IOP occurs before the age of 3 in primary congenital or infantile glaucoma or in the pediatric glaucomas associated with other ocular and/or systemic abnormalities.

## Epidemiology and Genetics

Glaucoma in the pediatric age group is heterogeneous. Isolated congenital glaucoma, which accounts for approximately 50%–70% of the congenital glaucomas, occurs much less frequently than primary adult glaucoma, and primary infantile glaucoma is believed to be rare. Of pediatric glaucoma cases, 60% are diagnosed by the age of 6 months and 80% within the first year of life. Approximately 65% of patients are male, and involvement is bilateral in 70% of all cases.

Although some pedigrees suggest an autosomal dominant inheritance, more patients show a recessive pattern with incomplete or variable penetrance and possibly multifactorial inheritance. Some types of juvenile glaucoma that have an autosomal dominant inheritance pattern have been mapped to chromosome 1q21–31. Some cases of primary congenital glaucoma have been associated with chromosomal rearrangement. The natural history of this disorder is variable. Prior to effective surgical therapy, the worst cases of the disease almost always resulted in blindness.

Some patients with congenital, infantile, or juvenile glaucoma may also have Axenfeld-Rieger syndrome, aniridia, or a multisystem genetic disorder. All pediatric patients with glaucoma and adults who had glaucoma in childhood should be evaluated by a geneticist for counseling purposes.

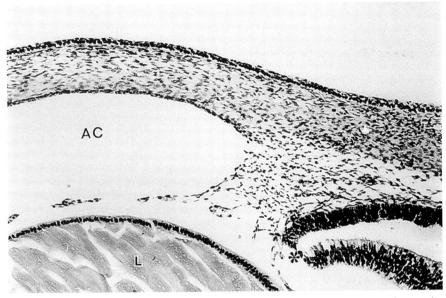

FIG VI-1—Light micrograph of the eye of an 11-week fetus in meridional section. The angular region is poorly defined at this stage and is occupied by loosely arranged, spindle-shaped cells. Schlemm's canal is unrecognizable, and ciliary muscles and ciliary processes are not yet formed; the latter are derived from neural ectodermal fold *(asterisk)*. Corneal endothelium appears continuous with cellular covering of primitive iris. *AC,* Anterior chamber. *L,* Lens. (Original magnification ×230.) (Reproduced with permission from Tripathi RC, Tripathi BJ. Functional anatomy of the anterior chamber angle. In: Tasman W, Jaeger EA, eds. *Duane's Foundations of Clinical Ophthalmology.* Philadelphia: Lippincott; 1991.)

## Pathophysiology

Figure VI-1 shows the normal development of the structures discussed here at 11 weeks. Because histopathologic findings in infantile glaucoma vary, many theories of pathogenesis have been proposed, which fall into two main groups. Some investigators have proposed that a cellular or membranous abnormality in the trabecular meshwork is the primary pathologic mechanism. This abnormality is described as either an anomalous impermeable trabecular meshwork or a Barkan membrane covering the trabecular meshwork. Other investigators have emphasized a more widespread anterior segment anomaly, including abnormal insertion of the ciliary muscle.

While the exact mechanism of primary infantile glaucoma remains unproven, there is little doubt that the disease represents a developmental anomaly of the angle structures. Many of its features suggest a developmental arrest in the late embryonic period. See also BCSC Section 2, *Fundamentals and Principles of Ophthalmology,* Part 2, Embryology.

## Clinical Features

Characteristic findings of infantile glaucoma include the classic triad of presenting symptoms in the newborn: *epiphora, photophobia,* and *blepharospasm.* Diagnosis of infantile glaucoma depends on careful clinical evaluation, including IOP measurement, measurement of corneal diameter, gonioscopy, measurement of axial length by ultrasonography, and ophthalmoscopy.

External eye examination may reveal buphthalmos with corneal enlargement greater than 12 mm in diameter during the first year of life. (The normal horizontal corneal diameter is 9.5–10.5 mm in full-term newborns and smaller in premature newborns.) Corneal edema may range from mild haze to dense opacification of the corneal stroma because of elevated IOP. Corneal edema is present in 25% of affected infants at birth and in more than 60% by the sixth month. Tears in Descemet's membrane called *Haab's striae* may occur acutely as a result of corneal stretching; these are typically oriented horizontally or concentric to the limbus.

Reduced visual acuity may occur as a result of optic atrophy, corneal clouding, astigmatism, amblyopia, cataract, lens dislocation, or retinal detachment. Amblyopia may be caused by the corneal opacity itself or by refractive error. The enlargement of the eye causes myopia, while tears in Descemet's membrane can cause a large astigmatism. Appropriate measures to prevent or treat amblyopia should be initiated as early as possible.

It is possible for the clinician to measure the IOP in some infants under age 6 months without general anesthesia or sedation by performing the measurement while the infant is feeding or asleep following feeding. However, critical evaluation of infants requires an examination under anesthesia. Most general anesthetic agents and sedatives lower IOP. In addition, infants may become dehydrated in preparation for general anesthesia, also reducing the IOP. As anesthesia becomes deeper, IOP falls. The only exception to this rule is ketamine, which may raise IOP. The normal IOP in an infant under anesthesia may range from 10 to 20 mm Hg, depending on the tonometer. A significant IOP elevation may occur in one eye only in 25%–30% of cases.

Gonioscopy under anesthesia, using a direct gonioscopic lens, is recommended. In isolated childhood glaucoma the anterior chamber is characteristically deep with normal iris structure. Findings include a high and flat iris insertion, absence of angle recess, peripheral iris hypoplasia, tenting of the peripheral iris pigment epithelium, and thickened uveal trabecular meshwork. The angle is typically open with a high insertion of the iris root that forms a scalloped line as a result of abnormal tissue with a shagreened, glistening appearance. This tissue holds the peripheral iris anteriorly. The angle is usually avascular, but loops of vessels from the major arterial circle may be seen above the iris root.

The normal anterior chamber angle in childhood is different from the adult angle. Many of the findings listed above are nonspecific, and it may be difficult to distinguish the gonioscopic findings in infantile glaucoma from a normal infant angle. If corneal edema prevents an adequate view of the angle, the epithelium may be removed with a scalpel blade or a cotton-tipped applicator soaked in 70% alcohol to improve visibility.

Visualization of the optic disc may be facilitated by using a direct ophthalmoscope and a direct gonioscopic or fundus lens on the cornea. The optic nerve head of a normal infant is pink with a small physiologic cup. Glaucomatous cupping in childhood resembles the cupping in adulthood, with preferential loss of neural tissue in the superior and inferior poles. In childhood the scleral canal enlarges in response to elevated IOP, causing enlargement of the cup. Cupping may be reversible if IOP is lowered, and progressive cupping indicates poor control of IOP.

Photographic documentation of the optic disc is recommended. Ultrasonography may be useful in documenting progression of glaucoma by recording increasing axial length. Increase in axial length may be reversible following reduction of IOP.

## Differential Diagnosis

Many other conditions with similar features are included in the differential diagnosis of infantile glaucoma (Table VI-1). Excessive tearing may be caused by an obstruction of the lacrimal drainage system. Ocular abnormalities associated with enlarged corneas include X-linked congenital megalocornea without glaucoma. Tears in

TABLE VI-1

DIAGNOSTIC CONSIDERATIONS FOR
SYMPTOMS AND SIGNS OF INFANTILE GLAUCOMA

***Excessive tearing***
  Nasolacrimal duct obstruction
  Corneal epithelial defect or abrasion
  Conjunctivitis

***Corneal enlargement or apparent enlargement***
  X-linked megalocornea
  High myopia
  Exophthalmos
  Shallow orbits (e.g., craniofacial dysostoses)

***Corneal clouding***
  Birth trauma
  Inflammatory corneal disease
  Congenital hereditary corneal dystrophies
  Corneal malformations (dermoid tumors, sclerocornea)
  Keratomalacia
  Metabolic disorders with associated corneal abnormalities (mucopolysaccharidoses, corneal lipidosis, cystinosis, and von Gierke disease)
  Skin disorders affecting the cornea (congenital ichthyosis and congenital dyskeratosis)
  Optic nerve abnormalities (optic nerve pit, optic nerve coloboma, optic nerve hypoplasia, physiologic cupping)

Descemet's membrane resulting from birth trauma, often associated with forceps-assisted deliveries, are usually vertical or oblique. Corneal opacification and clouding have many possible causes:

□ Birth trauma

□ Dysgeneses (Peters anomaly and sclerocornea)

□ Dystrophies (congenital hereditary endothelial dystrophy and posterior polymorphous dystrophy)

□ Choristomas (dermoid and dermislike choristoma)

□ Intrauterine inflammation (congenital syphilis and rubella)

□ Inborn errors of metabolism (mucopolysaccharidoses and cystinosis)

□ Keratomalacia

□ Skin disorders that affect the cornea (congenital ichthyosis and congenital dyskeratosis)

## Long-term Prognosis and Follow-up

Medications have limited long-term value for congenital and infantile glaucoma in most cases, and the preferred therapy is surgical. The initial procedures of choice are goniotomy if the cornea is clear and trabeculotomy ab externo if the cornea is hazy. The success rates are similar for both procedures. Trabeculectomy and shunt procedures should be reserved for those cases where goniotomy or trabeculotomy has failed.

Beta-adrenergic antagonists, alpha$_2$ agonists, or carbonic anhydrase inhibitors may be used as temporizing therapy prior to surgery to control IOP and help clear a cloudy cornea. These drugs must be used with caution and at doses appropriate for the child's weight to prevent systemic side effects. The parents should be instructed in particular to occlude the nasolacrimal drainage system for at least 2 minutes immediately after administering topical beta-adrenergic antagonists or alpha$_2$ agonists and to be alert for apnea and hypotension. Young children on carbonic anhydrase inhibitors require assessment for possible acidosis, hypokalemia, and feeding problems.

Long-term prognosis has greatly improved with the development of effective surgical techniques, particularly for patients who are asymptomatic at birth and present with onset of symptoms before 24 months of age. When symptoms are present at birth or when the disease is diagnosed after 24 months of age, the outlook for surgical control of IOP is more guarded. Even patients whose IOP is usually controlled by surgery may experience late complications such as amblyopia, corneal scarring, strabismus, anisometropia, cataract, lens subluxation, susceptibility of an eye with a thinned sclera to trauma, and recurrent glaucoma in the affected or unaffected eye many years later.

## Developmental Glaucomas with Associated Anomalies

Glaucoma may be associated with other ocular abnormalities, including the following conditions:

□ Microphthalmos

□ Corneal anomalies (microcornea, cornea plana, sclerocornea)

□ Anterior segment dysgenesis (Axenfeld-Rieger syndrome and Peters syndrome)

□ Aniridia

□ Lens anomalies (dislocation, microspherophakia)

□ Persistent hyperplastic primary vitreous

Glaucoma may occur in multisystem syndromes.

Developmental glaucoma with either an open or a closed angle may be associated with other anomalies. Some important anomalies include syndromes with known chromosomal abnormalities, systemic disorders of unknown etiology, and ocular congenital disorders. Glaucomas associated with congenital anomalies are summarized in Table VI-2 on pp 128–129.

A number of systemic disorders are also associated with pediatric glaucoma, including the following:

□ Sturge-Weber syndrome

□ Neurofibromatosis

□ Marfan syndrome

□ Homocystinuria

□ Weill-Marchesani syndrome

With Sturge-Weber syndrome and neurofibromatosis in particular, upper eyelid involvement is associated with an increased risk of glaucoma. A number of these conditions have ocular findings similar to primary infantile glaucoma; in others, the glaucoma is secondary.

Secondary glaucoma may develop in infants and children from any cause seen in adults: trauma, inflammation, retinopathy of prematurity with secondary angle-closure glaucoma, lens-induced glaucoma, corticosteroid-induced glaucoma, pigmentary glaucoma, and glaucoma secondary to intraocular tumors. Retinoblastoma, juvenile xanthogranuloma, and medulloepithelioma are some of the intraocular tumors known to lead to secondary glaucoma in infants and children. Rubella and congenital cataract are also important associated conditions. Clinicians now realize that children often develop glaucoma within 3 years following surgery for congenital cataract.

Higginbotham EJ, Lee DA, eds. *Management of Difficult Glaucoma: A Clinician's Guide.* Boston: Blackwell Scientific Publications; 1994.

Isenberg SJ, ed. *The Eye in Infancy.* 2nd ed. St Louis: Mosby; 1994.

Lee DA, ed. New developments in glaucoma. *Ophthalmol Clin North Am.* Philadelphia: Saunders; 1995;8:2.

TABLE VI-2

ANOMALIES ASSOCIATED WITH CHILDHOOD GLAUCOMAS

### Glaucoma associated with systemic congenital syndromes, with reported chromosomal abnormalities

Trisomy 21 (Down syndrome, trisomy G syndrome)

Mental deficiency, short stature, cardiac anomalies, hypotonia, atypical facies

Trisomy 13 (Patau syndrome)

Mental retardation, deafness, heart disease, motor seizures

Trisomy 18 (Edwards syndrome, trisomy E syndrome)

Low-set ears, high-arched hard palate, ventricular septal defects, rocker-bottom feet, short sternum, hypertonia

Turner (XO/XX) syndrome

Short stature, postadolescent females with sexual infantilism, webbed neck, mental retardation, congenital deafness, multiple systemic anomalies

### Glaucoma associated with systemic congenital disorders

Lowe (oculocerebrorenal) syndrome

X-linked recessive disease, mental retardation, renal rickets, aminoaciduria, hypotonia, acidemia, cataracts

Stickler syndrome (hereditary progressive arthro-ophthalmopathy)

Autosomal dominant connective tissue dysplasia; ocular, orofacial, and generalized skeletal abnormalities with high myopia; open-angle glaucoma; cataracts; vitreoretinal degeneration; retinal detachment

Zellweger (cerebrohepatorenal) syndrome

Congenital autosomal recessive syndrome, abnormal facies, cerebral dysgenesis, hepatic interstitial fibrosis, polycystic kidneys, central nervous system abnormalities
*Ocular findings:* nystagmus, corneal clouding, cataracts, retinal vascular and pigmentary abnormalities, optic nerve head lesions

Hallermann-Streiff syndrome (dyscephalic mandibulo-oculofacial syndrome, François dyscephalic syndrome)

Micrognathia, dwarfism, microphthalmos, cataract, aniridia, optic atrophy

Rubinstein-Taybi (broad-thumb) syndrome

Mental and motor retardation, typical congenital skeletal deformities of large thumbs and first toes
*Ocular findings:* bushy brows, hypertelorism, epicanthus, anti-mongoloid slant of eyelids, hyperopia, strabismus

Oculodentodigital dysplasia (Meyer-Schwickerath and Weyers syndrome)

Autosomal dominant inheritance, hypoplastic dental enamel, microdontia, bilateral syndactyly, thin nose, microcornea, microphthalmos

Prader-Willi syndrome

Chromosome 15 deletion, muscular hypotonia, hypogonadism, obesity, mental retardation
*Ocular findings:* ocular albinism, congenital ectropion uveae, iris stromal hypoplasia, angle abnormalities

Cockayne syndrome

Autosomal recessive disorder, dwarfism, mental retardation, progressive wasting, "birdlike" facies
*Ocular findings:* retinal degeneration, cataracts, corneal exposure, blepharitis, nystagmus, hypoplastic irides, irregular pupils

Fetal alcohol syndrome

Teratogenic effects of alcohol during gestation, facial abnormalities, mental retardation, anterior segment involvement resembling Axenfeld-Rieger syndrome and Peters anomaly, optic nerve hypoplasia

TABLE VI-2

ANOMALIES ASSOCIATED WITH CHILDHOOD GLAUCOMAS (continued)

### Glaucoma associated with ocular congenital disorders

Congenital ectropion uveae
Congenital corneal staphyloma
Cornea plana
Iridoschisis
Megalocornea
Microcoria
Microcornea
Microphthalmos
Morning glory syndrome
Persistent hyperplastic primary vitreous (PHPV)
Retinopathy of prematurity
Sclerocornea

Shields MB. *Textbook Of Glaucoma.* 4th ed. Baltimore: Williams & Wilkins; 1997.

Stamper RL, Lieberman MF, Drake MV, eds. *Becker-Shaffer's Diagnosis and Therapy of the Glaucomas.* 7th ed. St Louis: Mosby; 1999.

Tasman W, Jaeger EA, eds. *Duane's Clinical Ophthalmology.* Philadelphia: Lippincott; 1998.

# CHAPTER VII

# Medical Management of Glaucoma

Two decisions arise in choosing an appropriate glaucoma therapy: when to treat and how to treat. The risks of therapy must always be weighed against the anticipated benefits.

Primary angle-closure and infantile glaucoma are treated as soon as the diagnosis is made. Open-angle glaucoma is treated when damage to the optic nerve has been demonstrated in the form of progressive pathologic cupping and/or characteristic visual field defects, or when IOP is elevated to an extent that it is likely to cause damage to the optic nerve.

A patient with early open-angle glaucoma is difficult to distinguish from a glaucoma suspect. Since the latter has a relatively small risk of ultimate ocular damage, the decision of when to treat the glaucoma suspect who has not demonstrated actual nerve damage remains controversial. The Ocular Hypertension Treatment Study currently under way is attempting to determine whether medical reduction of IOP can prevent or delay the onset of glaucomatous damage in ocular hypertensive subjects (see Table IV-2). Most authorities agree that treatment of the glaucoma suspect should be limited to those patients with a high risk of damage to the optic nerve. Such patients may have risk factors that include elevated IOP, African-American descent, a positive family history of glaucoma, and asymmetric or suspicious cupping.

The goal of currently available glaucoma therapy is to preserve visual function by lowering IOP below a level that is likely to produce further damage to the nerve. The treatment regimen that achieves this goal with the lowest risk, fewest side effects, and least disruption of the patient's life should be the one employed. The so-called target pressure goal should actually be a range with an upper IOP limit that is unlikely to lead to further damage of the nerve in a given patient.

The more advanced the glaucomatous process on initial presentation, the lower the target pressure generally needs to be to prevent further progression. An initial reduction in the IOP of 20%–30% from baseline is suggested, but those patients who have progressive normal-tension glaucoma may require a decrease of at least 30% from baseline. *The target pressure range needs to be reassessed or changed as comparisons of IOP fluctuations, optic nerve changes, and/or visual field progression dictate.*

The anticipated benefits of any therapeutic regimen should justify the risks, and regimens associated with substantial side effects should be reserved for patients with a high probability of progressive visual loss. For example, it is reasonable to expose a patient to the side effects of systemic carbonic anhydrase inhibitors (CAIs) when significant damage to the visual field and optic nerve has occurred and the elevated IOP is not controlled by less toxic medications. When progressive visual field loss or cupping has not been established, however, the physician should exercise caution in subjecting a patient to the risk of the significant side effects of these agents.

The interrelationship between medical and surgical therapy is also complex. The treatment of pupillary-block angle-closure glaucoma and infantile glaucoma is primarily surgical, either laser or incisional, with medical therapy taking a secondary role. Initial treatment of primary open-angle glaucoma has commonly been medical, with surgery undertaken only if medical treatment fails or is not well tolerated. However, this assumption is currently under study; in some cases, initial surgery may prove more beneficial. Surgical therapy is discussed in detail in the following chapter.

> The Advanced Glaucoma Intervention Study (AGIS): 4. Comparison of treatment outcomes within race: seven-year results. *Ophthalmology.* 1998;105:1146–1164.

> The Advanced Glaucoma Intervention Study (AGIS): 7. The relationship between control of intraocular pressure and visual field deterioration. *Am J Ophthalmol.* 2000;130: 429–440.

> Lichter PR, Musch DC, Gillespie BW, et al. Interim clinical outcomes in the Collaborative Initial Glaucoma Treatment Study comparing initial treatment randomized to medications or surgery. *Ophthalmology.* 2001;108:1943–1953.

Treatment of secondary glaucoma is comparable to treatment of the primary glaucoma that it most closely resembles. In general, therapy should progress from the lowest risk to the higher risk, and then only when the initial treatments fail to reach target pressures and there is significant risk of progression. The efficacy of the therapeutic regimen should always be reevaluated periodically. Specifically, a one-eyed therapeutic trial should be considered for assessing efficacy of new medications, while a reverse therapeutic trial can also be performed to assess existing regimens.

## Medical Agents

Ocular hypotensive agents are divided into several groups based on chemical structure and pharmacologic action. The groups of agents in common clinical use include

- Beta-adrenergic antagonists (nonselective and selective)
- Parasympathomimetic (miotic) agents, including cholinergic and anticholinesterase agents
- Carbonic anhydrase inhibitors (oral, topical)
- Adrenergic agonists (nonselective and selective alpha$_2$ agonists)
- Prostaglandin analogues–hypotensive lipids
- Combination medications
- Hyperosmotic agents

The actions and side effects of the various glaucoma medications are listed in Table VII-1, along with dosage information and other concerns. The reader is referred back to this table throughout the discussions in this chapter. BCSC Section 2, *Fundamentals and Principles of Ophthalmology,* discusses and illustrates the mechanisms of action of these medications in Part 5, Ocular Pharmacology.

> Netland PA, Allen RC, eds. *Glaucoma Medical Therapy: Principles and Management.* Ophthalmology Monograph 13. San Francisco: American Academy of Ophthalmology; 1999.

TABLE VII-1

## Glaucoma Medications

| CLASS/COMPOUND | BRAND NAME | STRENGTHS | DOSAGE | METHOD OF ACTION | IOP DECREASE | SIDE EFFECTS OCULAR | SIDE EFFECTS SYSTEMIC | COMMENTS, INCLUDING TIME TO PEAK EFFECT AND WASHOUT |
|---|---|---|---|---|---|---|---|---|
| **Beta-adrenergic antagonists (beta blockers)** | | | | | | | | |
| *Nonselective* | | | | | | | | |
| Timolol maleate | Timoptic XE<br>Timoptic<br>Ocudose<br>Timolol gel | 0.25, 0.5%<br>0.25, 0.5%<br>0.25, 0.5%<br>0.5% | qd<br>qd, bid<br>qd, bid<br>qd | Decrease aqueous production | 20%–30% | Blurring, irritation, corneal anesthesia, punctate keratitis, allergy | Bradycardia, heart block, bronchospasm, decreased libido, CNS depression, mood swings | May be less effective if patient on systemic beta blockers, short-term escape, long-term drift<br>Peak: 2–3 hours<br>Washout: 1 month |
| Timolol hemihydrate | Betimol | 5.12 mg/ml | qd, bid | Same as above | Same as above | Same as above | Same as above | Less expensive |
| Levobunolol | Betagan | 0.25, 0.5% | qd, bid | Same as above | Same as above | Same as above | Same as above | Peak: 2–6 hours |
| Metipranolol | OptiPranolol | 0.3% | bid | Same as above | Same as above | Same as above | Same as above | Report of iritis<br>Peak: 2 hours |
| Carteolol hydrochloride | Ocupress | 1.0% | qd, bid | | | | Intrinsic sympathomimetic | May have less effect on nocturnal pulse, blood pressure<br>Peak: 4 hours<br>Washout: 1 month |
| *Selective* | | | | | | | | |
| Betaxolol | Betoptic (S) | 0.25% | bid | Same as above | 15%–20% | Same as above | Fewer pulmonary complications | Peak: 2–3 hours<br>Washout: 1 month |
| **Adrenergic agonists** | | | | | | | | |
| *Nonselective* | | | | | | | | |
| Epinephrine | Epifrin | 0.25, 0.5, 1.0, 2.0% | bid | Improve aqueous outflow | 15%–20% | Irritation, conjunctival hyphema (rebound), eyelid retraction, mydriasis, adrenochrome deposits, follicular conjunctivitis (allergy), cystoid macular edema in aphakia, pseudophakia | Hypertension, headaches, extra systoles | Peak: variable, initial IOP rise followed by reduction lasting 12–24 hours<br>Washout: 7–14 days |

| CLASS/COMPOUND | BRAND NAME | STRENGTHS | DOSAGE | METHOD OF ACTION | IOP DECREASE | SIDE EFFECTS OCULAR | SIDE EFFECTS SYSTEMIC | COMMENTS, INCLUDING TIME TO PEAK EFFECT AND WASHOUT |
|---|---|---|---|---|---|---|---|---|
| Dipivefrin HCl | Propine | 0.1% | bid | Same as above | Same as above | Same as above | Pro-drug makes systemic effects less likely | Peak/washout: same as epinephrine |
| **Alpha₂-adrenergic agonists** | | | | | | | | |
| *Selective* | | | | | | | | |
| Apraclonidine HCl | Iopidine | 0.5, 1.0% | bid, tid | Decrease aqueous production, decrease episcleral venous pressure | 20%–30% | Irritation, ischemia, allergy, eyelid retraction, conjunctival blanching, follicular conjunctivitis, puritis, dermatitis, ocular ache, photopsia, miosis | Hypotension, vasovagal attack, dry mouth and nose, fatigue | Useful in pre- or postlaser or cataract surgery, tachyphylaxis Peak: <1–2 hours Washout: 7–14 days |
| *Highly selective* | | | | | | | | |
| Brimonidine tartrate 0.2% | Alphagan | 0.2% | bid, tid | Decrease aqueous production, increase uveoscleral outflow | 20%–30% | Blurring, foreign body sensation, eyelid edema, dryness, less ocular sensitivity/allergy than Iopidine | Headache, fatigue, hypotension, insomnia, depression, syncope, dizziness, anxiety | Primary adrenergic agent in current use, highly alpha₂ selective Peak: 2 hours Washout: 7–14 days |
| Brimonidine tartrate in purite 0.15% | Alphagan P | 0.15% | bid, tid | Same as above | Same as above | Same except less allergy than Alphagan | Same except less fatigue and depression than Alphagan | Same as above |
| **Parasympathomimetic (miotic) agents** | | | | | | | | |
| *Cholinergic agonists (direct acting)* | | | | | | | | |
| Pilocarpine HCl | Isopto Carpine | 0.2%–10.0% | bid–qid | Increase trabecular outflow | 15%–25% | Posterior synechiae, keratitis, miosis, brow ache, cataract growth, angle-closure potential, myopia, retinal tear/detachment, dermatitis, change in retinal sensitivity, color vision changes | Increased salivation, increased secretion (gastric), abdominal cramps | Exacerbation of cataract effect, more effective in lighter irides Peak: 1½–2 hours Washout: 48 hours |
| | Pilocar | 0.5, 1.0, 2.0, 3.0, 4.0, 6.0% | bid–qid | | | | | |

continued

TABLE VII-1

GLAUCOMA MEDICATIONS (continued)

| CLASS/COMPOUND | BRAND NAME | STRENGTHS | DOSAGE | METHOD OF ACTION | IOP DECREASE | SIDE EFFECTS OCULAR | SIDE EFFECTS SYSTEMIC | COMMENTS, INCLUDING TIME TO PEAK EFFECT AND WASHOUT |
|---|---|---|---|---|---|---|---|---|
| Pilocarpine gel | Pilopine Gel HS | 4.0% | qhs | Increase trabecular outflow | 15%–25% | Same as above | Same as above | Same as above Peak: 2–3 hours Washout: 48 hours |
| Carbachol* | Isopto Carbachol | 1.5, 3.0% | bid, tid | Same as above | 15%–25% | May be useful in patients with pilocarpine sensitivity | | Intraoperative carbachol useful to lower IOP |
| *Anticholinesterase agents (indirect acting)* | | | | | | | | |
| Demecarium bromide | Humorsol | 0.125, 0.25% | qd, bid | Same as above | 15%–25% | Intense miosis, iris pigment cyst, myopia, cataract, retinal detachment, angle closure, punctal stenosis, pseudopemphigoid | Same as pilocarpine, more gastrointestinal difficulties | Increased inflammation with ocular surgery; may be helpful in aphakia, anesthesia risks (prolonged recovery); useful in eyelid-lash lice, postoperative cataract surgery |
| **Carbonic anhydrase inhibitors** | | | | | | | | |
| *Oral* | | | | | | | | |
| Acetazolamide | Diamox Diamox Sequels | 62.5, 125, 250 mg 500 mg | bid–qid qd, bid | Decrease aqueous production | 15%–20% | None | Poor tolerance of carbonated beverages, acidosis, depression, malaise, hirsutism, flatulence, paresthesias, numbness, lethargy, blood dyscrasias, diarrhea, weight loss, renal stones, loss of libido, bone marrow depression, hypokalemia, cramps, anorexia, altered taste, increased serum urate, enuresis | Sulfa allergy, caution to patients susceptible to ketoacidosis, hepatic insufficiency |
| Acetazolamide (parenteral) | Diamox | 500 mg 5–10 mg/kg | Usually ≤1qd q6–8 hrs | Same as above | Same as above | Same as above | Same as above | Same as above |

| CLASS/ COMPOUND | BRAND NAME | STRENGTHS | DOSAGE | METHOD OF ACTION | IOP DECREASE | SIDE EFFECTS | | COMMENTS, INCLUDING TIME TO PEAK EFFECT AND WASHOUT |
|---|---|---|---|---|---|---|---|---|
| | | | | | | OCULAR | SYSTEMIC | |
| Dichlorphenamide | Daranide | 50 mg | bid, tid | Same as above | Same as above | Same as above | Same as above | Same as above |
| Methazolamide | Neptazane | 25, 50, 100 mg | bid, tid | Same as above | Same as above | Same as above | Same as above | Same as above |
| *Topical* | | | | | | | | |
| Dorzolamide | Trusopt | 2.0% | bid, tid | Same as above | 15%–20% | Induced myopia, blurred vision, stinging, keratitis, conjunctivitis, dermatitis | Less likely to induce systemic effects of CAI, but may occur; bitter taste | Peak: 2–3 hours Washout: 48 hours |
| Brinzolamide | Azopt | 1% | bid, tid | Same as above | Same as above | Less stinging when compared to Trusopt | Same as above | Same as above |
| ***Hypotensive lipids*** | | | | | | | | |
| *Prostaglandin analogues* | | | | | | | | |
| Latanoprost | Xalatan | .005% | qd | Increase uveoscleral ouflow | 25%–32% | Increased pigmentation of iris and lashes, hypertrichiasis, blurred vision, keratitis, CME, anterior uveitis, conjunctival hyperemia | Flulike symptoms, joint/muscle pain, headache | ± IOP lowering effect with miotic Peak: 10–14 hours Washout: 4–6 weeks |
| Travoprost | Travatan | .004% | qd | Same as above | 25%–32% | Same as above | Same as above | Same as above |
| *Prostamides* | | | | | | | | |
| Bimatoprost | Lumigan | 0.03% | qd | Increase uveoscleral and trabecular outflow | 27%–33% | Same as above | Same as above | Same as above |
| *Decosanoids* | | | | | | | | |
| Unoprostone isopropyl | Rescula | 0.15% | bid | Increase trabecular outflow | 13%–18% | Same as above | Same as above | Peak: unknown Washout: unknown |

*continued*

*Also has indirect actions.

## TABLE VII-1

### GLAUCOMA MEDICATIONS (continued)

| CLASS/ COMPOUND | BRAND NAME | STRENGTHS | DOSAGE | METHOD OF ACTION | IOP DECREASE | SIDE EFFECTS OCULAR | SIDE EFFECTS SYSTEMIC | COMMENTS, INCLUDING TIME TO PEAK EFFECT AND WASHOUT |
|---|---|---|---|---|---|---|---|---|
| **Hyperosmotic agents** | | | | | | | | |
| Mannitol (parenteral) | Osmitrol | 5.25% soln | 2 g/kg body wt | Osmotic gradient dehydrates vitreous | | IOP rebound, increased aqueous flare | Urinary retention, headache, congestive heart failure, expansion of blood volume, diabetic complications, nausea, vomiting, diarrhea, electrolyte disturbance, renal failure | Caution in heart failure; may precipitate diabetic ketoacidosis; useful in acute increased IOP; isosorbide less nausea, vomiting |
| Glycerin (oral) | Osmoglyn | 50% soln | 4–7 oz | Same as above | | Similar to above | Can cause problems in diabetic patients; similar to above | |
| **Fixed combinations** | | | | | | | | |
| Timolol/ Dorzolamide | Cosopt (Timoptic/Trusopt) | 0.5%/2% | bid | Decrease aqueous production | 25%–30% | Same as nonselective oral beta blocker, topical CAI | Same as nonselective oral beta blocker, topical CAI | Peak: 2–3 hours Washout: 1 month |

## Beta-Adrenergic Antagonists (Beta Blockers)

Topical beta-blocking agents lower IOP by inhibiting cyclic aden~~~~ phate (cAMP) production in ciliary epithelium, thereby reducing ~~~~ secretion 20%–50% (2.5 ml/min to 1.9 ml/min), with a correspond~~~~ of 20%–30%. The effect of beta blockers on aqueous producti~~~~ 1 hour of installation and can be present for up to 4 weeks after di~~~~ systemic absorption occurs, a contralateral effect with lowering ~~~~ untreated eye can also be observed.

Beta blockers are additive in combination with miotics, adrenergic agonists, CAIs (both topical and systemic), and prostaglandin analogues. Combinations of beta blockers and nonselective adrenergic agonists are only slightly additive, whereas more effect can be expected when combined with an alpha$_2$ agonist. Approximately 10%–20% of the patients treated with topical beta blockers fail to respond with significant lowering of the IOP. It should be noted that if a patient is on systemic beta-blocker therapy, then the addition of a topical beta blocker may be significantly less effective. Extended use of beta blockers may reduce their effectiveness, as the response of beta receptors is affected by constant exposure to an agonist (long-term drift, tachyphylaxis). Similarly, receptor saturation (drug-induced upregulation of beta receptors) may occur within a few weeks, with loss of effectiveness (short-term escape).

Six topical beta-adrenergic antagonists are approved for use for the treatment of glaucoma in the United States: betaxolol, carteolol, levobunolol, metipranolol, timolol maleate, and timolol hemihydrate. All except betaxolol are noncardioselective beta$_1$ and beta$_2$ antagonists. Beta$_1$ activity is largely cardiac and beta$_2$ activity largely pulmonary. Since betaxolol is a selective beta$_1$ antagonist, it is significantly safer than the nonselective beta blockers when pulmonary, CNS, or other systemic conditions are considered. Betaxolol may be useful in patients with a history of bronchospastic disorders, although other therapies should be tried in lieu of betaxolol, as beta selectivity is only relative and not absolute, and some beta$_2$ effect can therefore remain. In general, the IOP-lowering effect of betaxolol is less than the nonselective beta-adrenergic antagonists.

Carteolol demonstrates intrinsic sympathomimetic activity, which means that, while acting as a competitive antagonist, it also causes a slight to moderate activation of receptors. Thus, even though carteolol produces beta-blocking effects, these may be tempered, reducing the effect on cardiovascular and respiratory systems. Carteolol may also be less likely to adversely effect the systemic lipid profile when compared with other beta blockers.

Both ocular and systemic side effects of beta-adrenergic antagonists are listed in Table VII-1. They include bronchospasm, bradycardia, increased heart block, lowered blood pressure, reduced exercise tolerance, and CNS depression. Diabetic patients may experience reduced glucose tolerance and masking of hypoglycemic signs and symptoms. Abrupt withdrawal of ocular beta blockers can exacerbate symptoms of hyperthyroidism. Although betaxolol is somewhat less effective than the other beta-adrenergic antagonists in lowering intraocular pressure, it may be a safer alternative in some patients.

It is important to determine if the patient has ever had asthma prior to the prescription of a beta-blocking agent, which may induce severe bronchospasm in susceptible patients. The pulse should be measured and the beta blocker withheld if the pulse rate is slow or if more than first-degree heart block is present. Myasthenia gravis may be aggravated by these drugs.

Other side effects of beta blockers include lethargy, mood changes, depression, altered mentation, light-headedness, syncope, visual disturbance, corneal anesthesia, punctate keratitis, impotence, reduced libido, allergy, and alteration of serum lipids. This change in lipids may be less evident in patients using an agent with intrinsic sympathomimetic activity.

## Parasympathomimetic Agents

Parasympathomimetic agents, commonly called *miotics,* have been used in the treatment of glaucoma for more than 100 years. They are divided into two groups:

☐ Direct-acting cholinergic agonists

☐ Indirect-acting anticholinesterase agents

Direct-acting agents affect the motor end plates in the same way as acetylcholine, which is transmitted at postganglionic parasympathetic junctions, as well as at other autonomic, somatic, and central synapses. Indirect-acting agents inhibit the enzyme acetylcholinesterase, thereby prolonging and enhancing the action of naturally secreted acetylcholine. *Pilocarpine* is the most commonly prescribed direct-acting agent. *Carbachol* has both direct and indirect actions, although its primary mechanism is direct. The only indirect-acting agent still available is *demecarium bromide* (see Table VII-1).

Both direct- and indirect-acting agents reduce IOP by causing contraction of the ciliary muscle, which pulls the scleral spur to tighten the trabecular meshwork, increasing the outflow of aqueous humor. These agents can reduce the IOP by 15%–25%. The currently accepted indications for miotic therapy include chronic treatment of increased IOP in patients with at least some filtering angle and prophylaxis for angle-closure glaucoma prior to iridectomy.

The parasympathomimetic agents have been shown to reduce uveoscleral outflow in animals, and it is possible that this action may actually worsen the glaucoma if miotics are used in patients with little to no trabecular outflow, although theories on the effects on the uveoscleral outflow system in humans remain speculative. In addition, these agents cause the pupillary sphincter to contract (hence their common name, *miotics*), stimulate secretory activity in the lacrimal and salivary glands, and disrupt the blood–aqueous barrier. These actions have little bearing on the IOP-lowering effect, except in angle-closure glaucoma, where the mechanical action of the contracting pupillary sphincter may pull the iris away from the trabecular meshwork.

Miotic agents have been associated with retinal detachment in some patients; use of stronger direct-acting miotics as opposed to weaker miotic agents leads to increased risk. If possible, an alternate medication may be considered in patients with peripheral retinal disease that predisposes them to retinal detachment. In view of the plethora of other ocular hypotensive agents now available, miotic therapy has become less commonly employed in general.

Induced myopia resulting from ciliary muscle contraction is a side effect common to all cholinergic miotic agents. The short-acting drugs may produce varying refractive changes, especially in young patients. Brow ache may accompany the ciliary spasm, and the miosis interferes with vision in dim light and in patients with lens opacities.

Sustained-release pilocarpine membranes and gel minimize the pharmacologic side effects of pilocarpine, while decreasing the frequency of required dosing. The membrane form (Ocusert) contained a polymer "sandwich," which allowed for the slow release of pilocarpine over 1 week. Pilocarpine Ocuserts were not widely used and are no longer available.

The other sustained-release formulation, pilocarpine adsorbed to a polymer gel, is administered once daily at bedtime (pilocarpine gel). Although the IOP-lowering effect may last 24 hours in some patients, other individuals show loss of drug effect after 18–20 hours. Induced myopia and miosis are less prominent with the gel than with drops, but they may still interfere with vision. If the gel has not dissipated by morning, the patient may have blurred vision on awakening. Pilocarpine gel may be useful in some younger patients, in patients bothered by variable myopia or intense miosis, in older patients with lens opacities, and in patients who have difficulty complying with more frequent dosing regimens.

Indirect-acting miotics or the stronger direct-acting agents may induce a paradoxical angle closure, because contraction of the ciliary muscle leads to forward movement of the lens–iris diaphragm, an increase in the anteroposterior diameter of the lens, and a very miotic pupil. These effects may increase pupillary block. The miosis may be visually disabling in patients with a central lens opacity such as a posterior subcapsular cataract. However, the concomitant administration of an alpha-adrenergic agonist such as phenylephrine may cause a larger pupil without interfering with the reduction of IOP. Again, newer medications have replaced this combination.

The indirect-acting miotics are cataractogenic, and evidence suggests that the direct-acting agents may also be weakly cataractogenic. Indirect-acting miotics may induce generalized cataract formation in addition to anterior subcapsular opacity. They may also induce the formation of iris pigment epithelial cysts. The strong miotics may cause epiphora by both direct lacrimal stimulation and punctal stenosis. These agents may also cause ocular surface changes resulting in drug-induced pseudopemphigoid.

Reports of increased inflammation following surgery associated with the use of stronger miotics suggest that these agents should be discontinued prior to surgery. In addition, the anticholinesterase agents should be discontinued and other agents substituted at least 2–4 weeks prior to ocular surgery, because they cause increased bleeding during surgery and severe fibrinous iridocyclitis postoperatively. Because miotics can break down the blood–aqueous barrier, their use in treating uveitic glaucoma should be limited.

While direct-acting miotics rarely induce systemic side effects, indirect-acting medications may be responsible for systemic parasympathetic stimulation. Diarrhea, abdominal cramps, increased salivation, bronchospasm, and even enuresis may result. Pseudocholinesterase activity in the red blood cells is depressed for 6 weeks after cessation of eyedrops. Since cholinesterase is suppressed throughout the body, depolarization agents such as succinylcholine should be avoided while the patient is using these eyedrops and for 6 weeks after discontinuation.

Because of the potential for significant ocular and systemic side effects, indirect-acting parasympathomimetic agents are used less commonly than the direct-acting agents. Indeed, indirect-acting agents are usually reserved for treatment of glaucoma in aphakic and pseudophakic eyes when IOP is not controlled by less toxic agents and in phakic eyes when filtering surgery has failed.

## Carbonic Anhydrase Inhibitors

These agents decrease aqueous humor formation by direct antagonist activity upon ciliary epithelial carbonic anhydrase and perhaps, to a lesser extent, by producing a generalized acidosis. The latter effect is controversial. The enzyme carbonic anhydrase is also present in many other tissues, including corneal endothelium, iris, retinal pigment epithelium, brain, and kidney. Over 90% of the ciliary epithelial enzyme activity must be abolished to decrease aqueous production and lower IOP.

The systemic agents are most useful in acute situations (e.g., acute angle-closure glaucoma). They can be given orally, intramuscularly, and intravenously. Because of the side effects of the systemic carbonic anhydrase inhibitors, however, chronic therapy with these agents should be reserved for patients whose glaucoma cannot be controlled by alternative topical therapy.

Systemic acetazolamide and methazolamide are the oral CAI agents most commonly used; another agent in this group is dichlorphenamide (see Table VII-1). Methazolamide has a longer duration of action and is less bound to serum protein than acetazolamide. Methazolamide and sustained-release acetazolamide are the best tolerated of the systemic CAIs. Methazolamide is metabolized by the liver, thereby decreasing some of the risk of systemic side effects. Acetazolamide is not metabolized and is excreted in urine.

Side effects of systemic CAI therapy are usually dose related. Many patients develop paresthesias of the fingers or toes and complain of lassitude, loss of energy, and anorexia. Weight loss is common. Abdominal discomfort, diarrhea, loss of libido, impotence, and an unpleasant taste in the mouth, as well as severe mental depression, may also occur. There is an increased risk in formation of calcium oxylate and calcium phosphate renal stones. Because methazolamide has greater hepatic metabolism and causes less acidosis, it may be less likely to cause renal lithiasis than acetazolamide.

Since CAIs are chemically derived from sulfa drugs, they have similar allergic reactions and cross reactivity. Aplastic anemia is a rare but potentially fatal idiosyncratic reaction to CAIs. Thrombocytopenia and agranulocytosis can also occur. Although routine complete blood counts have been suggested, they are not predictive of this idiosyncratic reaction and not routinely recommended. Hypokalemia is a potentially serious complication that is especially likely when oral CAIs are used concurrently with another drug that causes potassium loss (e.g., a thiazide diuretic). Serum potassium should be monitored regularly in such patients.

Clearly, CAIs are potent medications with significant side effects. The lowest dose that reduces the IOP to an acceptable range should be used. Methazolamide is often effective in doses as low as 25–50 mg given two to three times daily. Acetazolamide may be started at 62.5 mg every 6 hours, and higher doses may be used, if tolerated. Sustained-release formulations such as Diamox Sequels may have fewer side effects.

Topical CAI agents are also available for chronic treatment of IOP elevation. Dorzolamide and brinzolamide are sulfonamide derivatives that reduce aqueous formation by direct inhibition of carbonic anhydrase in the ciliary body with fewer systemic side effects than the oral agents. Dorzolamide and brinzolamide are currently available for use three times daily, although reduction of IOP is only slightly greater when compared to twice-daily therapy. Both agents are equally efficacious and reduce IOP (monotherapy) by 14%–17%, perhaps not as great a reduction as the oral CAIs.

Common adverse effects of topical CAIs include bitter taste, blurred vision, and punctate keratopathy. Ocular surface irritation with dorzolamide may be a result of the relative greater acidity (lower pH) when compared with brinzolamide. Eyes with compromised endothelial cell function may also be at risk for corneal decompensation. The brinzolamide suspension may cause more blurring than the dorzolamide solution. Systemic lassitude is a side effect as well.

## Adrenergic Agonists

The nonselective adrenergic agonists epinephrine and dipivefrin increase conventional trabecular and uveoscleral outflow. The latter appears to be influenced by epinephrine-induced stimulation of prostaglandin synthesis. Interestingly, epinephrine-related agents may initially increase aqueous production; with chronic use, however, they decrease it. Adding nonselective adrenergic agonists to beta antagonists usually produces modest additional pressure lowering.

Epinephrine, a mixed alpha and beta agonist, and related compounds have less hypotensive effect in eyes with dark irides. The IOP-lowering effect begins at 1 hour and is maximal at 2–6 hours. Individual responses to epinephrine used as a single drug therapy may vary from a 10% to a 20% decrease in IOP. Tolerance, or *tachyphylaxis,* is common with long-term use, although in some individuals, epinephrine may become more effective over time. Additionally, many patients become intolerant in response to extraocular reactions.

Epinephrine salts used in the past for the treatment of glaucoma included hydrochloride, borate, and bitartrate. Epinephrine bitartrate had about one half the available epinephrine of an equivalent solution of its hydrochloride, or of borate salt, which was the least irritating of the three.

Dipivefrin is a *pro-drug* that is chemically transformed into epinephrine by esterase enzymes in the cornea. Dipivefrin has greater corneal penetration than epinephrine salt, and the activity of this drug prior to its alteration by the esterase enzymes is relatively low. These qualities give it two major advantages over epinephrine salt:

□ A lower topical concentration of dipivefrin has an intraocular effect similar to a higher dosage of epinephrine salt.

□ Therapeutic effectiveness in the eye can be achieved with fewer topical and systemic side effects.

Dipivefrin is tolerated by some patients who are allergic to epinephrine salt. Its effectiveness may be diminished, however, if an anticholinergic agent, which may prevent dipivefrin's cleavage and activation by corneal esterases, is added.

Table VII-1 lists potential ocular and systemic side effects of both epinephrine and dipivefrin. Important systemic side effects include headache, increased blood pressure, tachycardia, arrhythmia, and nervousness. Epinephrine causes adrenochrome deposits from oxidized metabolites in the conjunctiva, cornea, and lacrimal system, and it may stain soft contact lenses (Fig VII-1). The use of these agents often causes pupillary dilation as a consequence of alpha-agonist action that stimulates norepinephrine receptors, and it may precipitate or aggravate angle closure in susceptible individuals. Allergic blepharoconjunctivitis occurs in approximately 20% of patients over time. Cystoid macular edema may be precipitated or exacerbated in aphakic and pseudophakic eyes without intact posterior capsules. Since this maculopathy is usually reversible if recognized early, epinephrine or dipivefrin should be used with caution in these eyes. Rebound conjunctiva hyperemia is common when these drugs are discontinued. Although this condition is harmless, patients may be disturbed by the appearance and usually need reassurance.

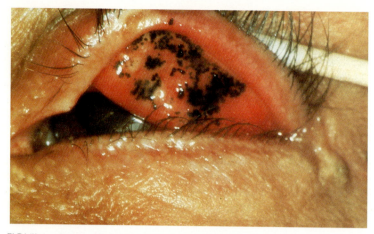

FIG VII-1—Conjunctiva with adrenochrome deposits following chronic epinephrine use. (Photograph courtesy of Elizabeth A. Hodapp, MD.)

*Alpha₂-adrenergic agonists* It has become evident that alpha₂ effects are desirable in glaucoma therapy. Alpha₁ effects include vasoconstriction, pupillary dilation, and eyelid retraction, while alpha₂ effects are primarily IOP reduction and possible neuroprotection. Apraclonidine and brimonidine are relatively selective alpha₂ agonists that have been developed for glaucoma therapy. Brimonidine is much more highly selective for the alpha₂ receptor than apraclonidine.

Apraclonidine hydrochloride (para-aminoclonidine) is an alpha₂-adrenergic agonist and a clonidine derivative that prevents release of norepinephrine at nerve terminals. It decreases aqueous production as well as episcleral venous pressure and improves trabecular outflow. However, its true ocular hypotensive mechanism is not fully understood. When administered pre- and postoperatively, the drug is effective in diminishing the acute IOP rise that follows argon laser iridectomy, argon laser trabeculoplasty, Nd:YAG laser capsulotomy, and cataract extraction. Apraclonidine hydrochloride may be effective for the short-term lowering of IOP, but development of topical sensitivity and tachyphylaxis often limits long-term use.

Brimonidine tartrate encounters less tachyphylaxis than apraclonidine in long-term use, and allergenicity such as follicular conjunctivitis and contact blepharitis-dermatitis is also lower (up to 40% for apraclonidine, less than 15% for brimonidine, and less than 10% for brimonidine P 0.15%). Cross sensitivity to brimonidine in patients with known hypersensitivity to apraclonidine is minimal. Brimonidine lowers IOP by decreasing aqueous production and increasing uveoscleral outflow. Similar to beta blockers, a peripheral mechanism may account for part of the IOP reduction from brimonidine 0.2%, as a single eye treatment trial for 1 week caused a statistically significant reduction of 1.2 mm Hg in the fellow eye.

Brimonidine's peak IOP reduction is approximately 26% (2 hours postdose). At peak it is comparable to a nonselective beta blocker and superior to the selective beta blocker betaxolol, although at trough (12 hours postdose) the reduction is only 14%–15%, or less effective than the nonselective beta blockers but comparable to betaxolol during the first 6–12 months of therapy. Long-term data demonstrate increased efficiency at trough compared with timolol. Brimonidine may also have potential neuroprotective properties, as shown in animal models of optic nerve and retinal injury, that are independent of IOP reduction. The proposed mechanism of neuroprotection is upregulation of a neurotrophin, basic fibroblast growth factor, and cellular regulatory genes that inhibit apoptosis.

Caution is recommended when using both apraclonidine or brimonidine in patients on a monoamine oxidase inhibitor (MAOI) or tricyclic antidepressant therapy. Use of these drugs concomitantly with beta blockers, antihypertensives, and cardiac glycosides (ophthalmic and systemic) also requires prudence. Although effective in acutely lowering the IOP in angle-closure glaucoma, these drugs may also induce vasoconstriction that can prolong iris sphincter ischemia and reduce the efficacy of concurrent miotics. Apraclonidine has a much greater affinity for alpha$_1$ receptors than does brimonidine and is therefore more likely to produce vasoconstriction in the eye. Brimonidine has been shown to not induce vasoconstriction in the posterior segment or optic nerve.

## Prostaglandin Analogues–Hypotensive Lipids

Prostaglandin (PG) analogues–hypotensive lipids are a relatively new class of ocular hypotensive agents. Currently, two PG analogues have been approved for clinical use: travoprost and latanoprost. Two other hypotensive lipids (bimatoprost and unoprostone isopropyl) have also been approved, but their effect on PGF receptors remains controversial. Unlike latanoprost and travoprost, which lower IOP by increasing uveoscleral outflow by 50%, bimatoprost decreases IOP by increasing uveoscleral outflow by 50% and increasing trabecular outflow by 25%–30%. Unoprostone appears to lower IOP by increasing trabecular outflow only.

Latanoprost and travoprost are pro-drugs that penetrate the cornea and become biologically active after being hydrolyzed by corneal esterase. Both latanoprost and travoprost reduce IOP by 25%–32%. Neither bimatoprost or unoprostone appears to be a pro-drug. Bimatoprost lowers IOP by 27%–33%; while unoprostone is less effective, lowering IOP 13%–18%. Latanoprost, travoprost, and bimatoprost are used once a day, while unoprostone is used twice daily.

An ocular side effect unique to this class of drugs is the darkening of the iris and periocular skin as a result of increased numbers of melanosomes (increased melanin content—melanogenesis) within the melanocytes. The risk of iris pigmentation correlates with baseline iris pigmentation. Blue irides may experience increased pigmentation in 10%–20% of eyes in the initial 18–24 months of therapy, whereas nearly 60% of eyes that are light brown, blue-green, or two-toned may experience increased pigmentation over the same time period. The long-term sequelae of this side effect is unknown. Other side effects reported in association with the use of a topical prostaglandin analogue–hypotensive lipid include conjunctival hyperemia, hypertrichosis of the eyelashes, exacerbations of underlying herpes keratitis, cystoid macular edema, and uveitis. The latter two side effects are more common in eyes with preexisting risk factors for either macular edema or uveitis. Studies to date have demonstrated that the incidence of these side effects varies among these four agents. Because bimatoprost, latanoprost, and travoprost reach peak effectiveness 10–14 hours after administration, bedtime application is recommended to maximize efficacy and decrease patient symptoms related to vascular dilatation.

travoprost
latanoprost
bimatoprost
unoprostone isopropyl

## Combined Medications

Medications that are combined and placed in a single bottle have the potential benefits of improved efficacy, convenience, and compliance, as well as reduced cost. Adrenergic agonists and parasympathomimetic agents (epinephrine and pilocarpine) have been available for many years as a combined agent. They are weakly additive in IOP-lowering effect, thus satisfying FDA guidelines that the fixed combination be more efficacious than either agent given alone. Epinephrine combined with a beta-blocker agent (Probeta = levobunolol plus dipivefrin 0.1%) is currently available in Canada. Beta blocker (timolol 0.5%) combined with miotic pilocarpine (either 2% or 4% concentration) is available for twice-daily therapy in Europe. Betanorm (beta-blocker metipranolol and pilocarpine) is available in many countries outside the United States.

Cosopt, the combination of a beta blocker (timolol 0.5%) and topical carbonic anhydrase inhibitor (dorzolamide 2%), has demonstrated similar efficacy compared with the two agents given separately: timolol 0.5% twice daily and Trusopt 2% given three times daily. The advantage of this combined therapy may be the convenience and lessened confusion of one bottle rather than two, which may increase the potential for greater compliance. However, the twice-daily dosing may create greater exposure to the potential beta-blocker systemic side effects, as beta blockers are generally equally effective when given only once daily. The ocular side effects are the same as for both drugs individually. The indications for this combined medication may be as a substitute for both a beta blocker and topical carbonic anhydrase inhibitor. If Cosopt is used as monotherapy, a monocular trial of timolol should be tried first. If timolol is effective in significantly lowering the IOP, then a monocular trial of dorzolamide should be used with timolol. An alternative trial could involve Cosopt in one eye twice daily and timolol in the opposite eye. It is important to prove that both the timolol component and the dorzolamide component each have an effect on IOP before choosing the combined medication.

## Hyperosmotic Agents

Hyperosmotic agents are used to control acute episodes of elevated IOP. Common hyperosmotic agents include oral glycerin and intravenous mannitol.

When given systemically, hyperosmotic agents lower the IOP by increasing the blood osmolality, which creates an osmotic gradient between the blood and the vitreous humor, drawing water from the vitreous cavity and reducing IOP. The larger the dose and the more rapid the administration, the greater the reduction in IOP because of the increased gradient. The substance distributed only in the extracellular water (e.g., mannitol) is more effective than a drug distributed in total body water (e.g., urea). When the blood–aqueous barrier is disrupted, the osmotic agent enters the eye faster than when the barrier is intact, thus reducing both the effectiveness of the drug and its duration of action.

Hyperosmotic agents are rarely administered for longer than a few hours because their effects are transient as a result of the rapid reequilibration of the osmotic gradient. They become less effective over time, and a rebound elevation in IOP may occur if the agent penetrates the eye and reverses the osmotic gradient.

Side effects of these drugs include headache, mental confusion, backache, and acute congestive heart failure and myocardial infarction. The rapid increase in extracellular volume and cardiac preload caused by hyperosmotic agents may precipitate or aggravate congestive heart failure. Intravenous administration is more likely than oral dosage to cause this problem. In addition, subdural and subarachnoid hemorrhages have been reported after treatment with hyperosmotic agents. Glycerin can produce hyperglycemia or even ketoacidosis in diabetic patients, since it is metabolized into sugar and ketone bodies.

## General Approach to Medical Treatment

### Open-Angle Glaucoma

The clinician should tailor therapy for open-angle glaucoma to the individual needs of the patient. As noted previously, a target IOP range is established as a goal. However, the effectiveness of therapy can only be established by careful repeated scrutiny of the patient's optic nerve and visual field status.

Characteristics of the medical agents available for the treatment of glaucoma are summarized in Table VII-1. The clinician making management decisions should keep efficacy and compliance in mind. Treatment is usually initiated with a single topical medication, unless the starting IOP is extremely high, in which case combination therapy may be indicated. A beta blocker is commonly the drug of choice for initial therapy, assuming there is no medical contraindication. However, because of potential systemic/ocular beta-blocker side effects, initiation with a selective alpha$_2$ agonist, topical CAI, or PG analogue can also be considered. Because of the variability of IOP, it is best (unless the IOP is extremely high) to test the medication in one eye until the effectiveness of therapy has been established. At that point, both eyes can be treated.

Patients should be taught how to space their medications and instructional charts should be given. It may be useful to coordinate the administration of medication with a part of the daily routine such as meals. Patients should be shown how to administer eyedrops properly. Eyedrops to be given at the same time should be separated by at least 5 minutes to prevent washout of the first by the second. Instructions on nasolacrimal occlusion or gentle eyelid closure to reduce the systemic effects from topical eye medications should be given. Teaching the patient to close the eyes for 1 full minute after instillation of the drop helps promote corneal penetration and reduce systemic absorption. An assistive drop device may be considered.

If one drug is not adequate to reduce IOP to the estimated desired safe level, another agent should be tried, preferably as a therapeutic trial in one eye. If no single agent controls the pressure, a combination of topical agents should be used. A beta blocker with an alpha$_2$ agonist, topical CAI, or PG analogue should be considered as second-line agents, and then miotic therapy followed by systemic CAI may be used. Clearly, when the individual is requiring three or more medications, compliance becomes more difficult and the potential for local ocular and systemic side effects increases.

Patients rarely associate systemic side effects with topical drugs and, consequently, seldom volunteer symptoms. The ophthalmologist must inquire about these symptoms. Communication with the primary care physician is important not only to let the family doctor know the potential side effects of antiglaucoma medication but also to discuss the interactions of any other systemic medications with the glaucoma process. Modification of systemic beta-blocker therapy for hypertension, for example, may affect glaucoma control. Physicians should be aware that compliance may decline as the complexity and expense of the medical regimen increase.

Patients with open-angle glaucoma require careful monitoring. IOP, while important, is only one factor, and optic nerve photographs or drawings and visual fields must be compared periodically to determine the stability of the disease (see Chapter III). The condition of the patient and the severity of the disease determine how often each of these parameters must be checked. If the cupping or visual field damage shows evidence of progression despite apparent control of acceptable IOP, other diseases should be considered (see discussion of normal-tension glaucoma in Chapter IV). Other possible explanations include an IOP level too high for the particular patient's optic nerve, IOP that may be spiking at times when the patient is not in the office, concomitant angle closure, and poor patient compliance.

## Angle-Closure Glaucoma

Medical treatment for acute angle-closure glaucoma is aimed at preparing the patient for laser iridectomy. The goals of medical treatment are to reduce IOP rapidly to prevent further damage to the optic nerve, to clear the cornea, to reduce intraocular inflammation, to allow pupillary constriction, and to prevent formation of posterior and peripheral anterior synechiae (see Chapter V). Treatment of chronic angle closure is the same as POAG, although miotics may induce a paradoxical increase in IOP if the angle is closed and the trabecular meshwork is nonfunctional.

CHAPTER VIII

# Surgical Therapy of Glaucoma

Surgical therapy of glaucoma is undertaken when medical therapy is not appropriate, not tolerated, not effective, or not properly utilized by a particular patient, and the glaucoma remains uncontrolled with either documented progressive damage or a very high risk of further damage. Surgery is usually the primary approach for infantile and pupillary-block glaucoma. The relative roles of medical and surgical intervention in the therapy of open-angle glaucoma remain the subject of an ongoing study, the Collaborative Initial Glaucoma Treatment Study (CIGTS). Surgery has traditionally been considered for open-angle glaucoma only when medical therapy has failed and is associated with long-term risks of bleb-associated problems, cataracts, and infection. Studies of trabeculectomy as initial therapy for glaucoma, however, suggest that there may be some advantages such as reduction of patient visits to the doctor and possibly better visual field preservation.

Migdal C, Gregory W, Hitchings R. Long-term functional outcome after early surgery compared with laser and medicine in open-angle glaucoma. *Ophthalmology.* 1994; 101:1651–1657.

Musch DC, Lichter PR, Guire KE, et al. The Collaborative Initial Glaucoma Treatment Study: study design, methods, and baseline characteristics of enrolled patients. *Ophthalmology.* 1999;106:653–662.

When surgery is indicated, the clinical setting must guide the selection of the appropriate procedure. Each of the many possible procedures is appropriate in specific conditions and clinical situations. Many different glaucoma surgical procedures are performed to lower IOP. Among these are trabeculectomy and its variations, nonpenetrating filtration procedures, glaucoma drainage tube implants, angle surgery for congenital glaucoma, and ciliary body ablation. Other procedures such as iridectomy and gonioplasty address the problems of aqueous access to the angle. For each condition it is necessary to understand the indications, contraindications, and preoperative evaluation necessary for surgical planning. Understanding of the pathophysiology of the disease, as discussed throughout this volume, is essential to generating an appropriate surgical plan.

Glaucoma surgery can be accomplished with laser or incisional surgical techniques. The discussion in this chapter follows a systematic approach to help the clinician in decision making. Each surgical procedure is described in terms of indications, contraindications, techniques, and complications and other considerations.

## Surgery for Open-Angle Glaucoma

Surgery is indicated in open-angle glaucoma when IOP cannot be maintained by nonsurgical therapies at a level considered low enough to prevent further pressure-related damage to the optic nerve or visual field loss. The glaucoma may be uncontrolled for various reasons:

☐ Maximal medical therapy fails to adequately reduce IOP

☐ The amount of medical therapy necessary to control IOP is not well tolerated or places the patient at unacceptable risk

☐ Optic nerve cupping or visual field loss is progressing despite apparent "adequate" reduction of IOP with medical therapy

☐ The patient cannot comply with the necessary medical regimen

### Laser Trabeculoplasty (LTP)

**Indications** Historically, the indication for LTP could be simply expressed as the following: a patient with glaucoma on maximum tolerated medical therapy who requires lower IOP and in whom the angle is open on gonioscopy. However, a multicenter study, the Glaucoma Laser Trial, investigated the role of initial LTP in POAG and found laser to be at least as effective as medications for the first 2 years (see discussion of this study below). At present, most clinicians still initiate some form of medical therapy before advancing to LTP, but it is not unreasonable to consider LTP as a next step in the management of glaucoma when a patient is taking one or more medications. Laser trabeculoplasty is sometimes considered as the initial therapy for primary open-angle glaucoma and perhaps other open-angle glaucomas as well. The question the surgeon must address is when in the course of glaucoma therapy is it appropriate to employ LTP, since the duration of efficacy appears limited in most patients.

The Glaucoma Laser Trial (GLT) Research Group conducted a multicenter, randomized clinical trial to assess the efficacy and safety of LTP as an alternative to treatment with topical medication in patients with newly diagnosed, previously untreated primary open-angle glaucoma. Within the first 2 years of follow-up, LTP as initial therapy appeared to be as effective as medication. However, more than half of eyes treated initially with laser required the addition of one or more medications to control IOP over the course of the study. Further, the medication protocols used in the study no longer resemble the medical regimens commonly employed for the treatment of POAG.

Many ophthalmologists believe it is premature to recommend LTP as an initial therapy until more long-term data are available. The patient should understand that LTP may postpone the need for conventional surgery or additional medications. However, as with all glaucoma therapy, patients should not assume that their glaucoma is cured by this procedure, and they should be reminded that their disease requires lifelong monitoring.

Glaucoma Laser Trial Research Group. The Glaucoma Laser Trial (GLT). 2. Results of argon laser trabeculoplasty versus topical medicines. *Ophthalmology.* 1990;97:1403–1413.

Glaucoma Laser Trial Research Group. The Glaucoma Laser Trial (GLT) and glaucoma laser trial follow-up study. 7. Results. *Am J Ophthalmol.* 1995;120:718–731.

Laser trabeculoplasty effectively reduces IOP in patients with primary open-angle glaucoma, pigmentary glaucoma, and exfoliation syndrome. Aphakic and pseudophakic eyes may respond less favorably than phakic eyes; therefore, LTP may be more effective before than after cataract surgery. IOP reduction does not seem to be diminished by subsequent cataract extraction. When effective, LTP is expected to lower IOP 20%–25%. The risk:benefit ratio is highly favorable for LTP; this procedure should be considered for most eyes not sufficiently responsive to medical therapy.

***Contraindications*** There are few contraindications to LTP in POAG when the angle is accessible. It works least effectively in patients with inflammatory glaucoma or with membranes in the angle or in young patients who have developmental defects. LTP can be tried in angle recession, but the underlying tissue alterations may cause it to be ineffective. Another relative contraindication of LTP is the lack of effect in the fellow eye. If the eye has advanced damage and high IOP, LTP is unlikely to achieve a low target IOP.

***Preoperative evaluation*** As with all ocular surgery, the preoperative evaluation for LTP should include a detailed medical and ocular history and a comprehensive eye examination. Particular attention must be paid to visual field examination, gonioscopy, and optic nerve evaluation. The angle must be open gonioscopically. The amount of pigment in the angle will help determine the laser settings for argon laser; a more pigmented angle responds to lower laser energy. While eyes require some visible pigment in the angle for effective argon laser trabeculoplasty, this may not be the case for selective laser trabeculoplasty, which is discussed below.

***Technique*** In the argon laser procedure, a 50-µm laser beam of 0.1 second duration is focused through a goniolens at the junction of the anterior unpigmented and the posterior pigmented edge of the trabecular meshwork (Fig VIII-1). Application to the posterior trabecular meshwork tends to produce inflammation, pigment dispersion, prolonged elevation of IOP, and PAS. The power setting (300–1000 mW) should be titrated to achieve the desired end point: blanching of the trabecular meshwork or production of a tiny bubble. If a large bubble appears, the power is reduced. As LTP was originally described, laser energy was applied to the entire circumference (360°) of the trabecular meshwork. Evidence suggests that many patients have a satisfactory IOP reduction with less risk of short-term pressure elevation when only one half of the circumference (180°) is treated, using approximately 40–50 applications.

The procedure with the diode laser is similar; a 75-µm laser beam is focused through a goniolens with a power setting of 600–1000 mW and duration of 0.02 second.

***Complications*** The most significant complication of laser trabeculoplasty is a transient rise in IOP, which occurs in approximately 20% of patients. IOP has been reported to reach 50–60 mm Hg and may cause additional damage to the optic nerve. This rise is less common when only 180° of the angle is treated per session.

IOP elevations are of particular concern in patients with advanced cupping. Rises in IOP are usually evident within the first 2–4 hours after treatment, and all patients should be monitored closely for this complication. The adjunctive use of topical apraclonidine 1% has been shown to blunt postoperative pressure elevation. This formulation was developed for acute use as prophylaxis with laser surgery.

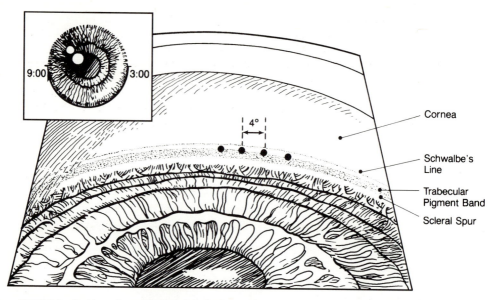

FIG VIII-1—Position of argon laser trabeculoplasty treatment in the trabecular meshwork. Inset shows 180° application of laser treatment. (After Solish AM, Kass MA. Laser trabeculoplasty. In: Waltman SR, Keates RH, Hoyt CS, eds. *Surgery of the Eye*. New York: Churchill Livingstone; 1988:1.)

Many surgeons use apraclonidine 0.5% or brimonidine 0.2% for prophylaxis against IOP spike even though these drugs were not investigated and do not have FDA-approved indications at these concentrations for this use. Other topical medications shown to blunt the IOP spikes include beta blockers, pilocarpine, and topical CAIs. Hyperosmotic agents, oral CAIs, and ice packs may be helpful in eyes with IOP spikes not responsive to topical medications.

Low-grade iritis may follow LTP. Some surgeons routinely treat with topical anti-inflammatory drugs for 1 week, while others use them only if inflammation develops. Other complications of LTP include the rare persistent elevation of IOP requiring filtering surgery, hyphema, and the formation of PAS.

***Results and long-term follow-up*** From 4 to 6 weeks should be allowed to evaluate the full effect of the first treatment before a decision is made about additional treatment. Approximately 80% of patients with medically uncontrolled open-angle glaucoma experience a drop in IOP for a minimum of 6–12 months following LTP. Longer-term data have shown that 50% of patients with an initial response maintain a significantly lower IOP 3–5 years after treatment. Success at 10 years approximates 30%. Highest success rates are seen in older patients with POAG and psueudoexfoliative glaucoma. Eyes with pigmentary glaucoma may show a good initial decrease in IOP, but with continued pigment shedding, this decrease may not be sustained.

Elevation of IOP may recur in some patients after months or even years of control. Additional laser treatment may be helpful in some patients, especially if the entire angle has not been treated previously. Retreatment of an angle that has been fully treated (approximately 80–100 spots over 360°) has a lower success rate and a higher complication rate than does primary treatment. If initial laser trabeculoplasty fails to bring IOP under control, a trabeculectomy should be considered.

The mechanism of action of LTP remains unclear, although outflow facility improves following successful trabeculoplasty. Histopathologic examination suggests that LTP may stimulate the growth of trabecular meshwork endothelial cells. Although the long-term implications of this finding remain unknown, it has been suggested that these stimulated cells may restore trabecular meshwork function.

Englert JA, Cox TA, Allingham RR, et al. Argon vs diode laser trabeculoplasty. *Am J Ophthalmol.* 1997;124:627–631.

Panek WC. Role of laser treatment in glaucoma. In: *Focal Points: Clinical Modules for Ophthalmologists.* San Francisco: American Academy of Ophthalmology; 1993: vol 11, no 1.

Ritch R, Shields MB, Krupin T, eds. *The Glaucomas.* 2nd ed. St Louis: Mosby; 1996.

Wise JB, Witter SL. Argon laser therapy for open-angle glaucoma: a pilot study. *Arch Ophthalmol.* 1979;97:319–322.

## Selective Laser Trabeculoplasty

Currently, this is an investigational procedure in which the laser targets intracellular melanin. Preliminary results suggest that the procedure is safe and effective with IOP results similar to those achieved with argon LTP. Preliminary evidence also suggests that this procedure may be repeated and still be effective with less risk of damage to the trabecular meshwork. Long-term studies are being conducted to clarify and validate these preliminary findings.

Latina MA, Sibayan SA, Shin DH, et al. Q-switched 532-nm Nd:YAG laser trabeculoplasty (selective laser trabeculoplasty): a multicenter, pilot, clinical study. *Ophthalmology.* 1998;105:2082–2090.

## Incisional Surgery for Open-Angle Glaucomas

Although incisional procedures to lower IOP are traditionally referred to as *filters,* it would be more correct physiologically and anatomically to refer to them as *fistulizing procedures.* This discussion will use the traditional terminology, which remains in widespread use. The goal of filtering surgery is to create a new pathway (fistula) for the bulk flow of aqueous humor from the anterior chamber through the surgical defect in the sclera into the subconjunctival and sub-Tenon's spaces. The filtering procedure most commonly used is guarded trabeculectomy. Full-thickness procedures have largely fallen into disuse because of the high complication rate, especially since the introduction of antifibrotic agents.

**Indications**   The indication for incisional surgery for glaucoma has been expressed as: "A patient with glaucoma on maximum tolerable medical therapy who has had maximal laser benefit and whose optic nerve function is failing or is likely to fail."

This statement raises several important considerations. The presence of glaucoma and a high probability of optic nerve damage is a clear indication. With the potential complications of glaucoma surgery, however, it is not reasonable to perform a trabeculectomy in an ocular hypertensive eye with a low risk of developing damage. In less clearcut situations—for example, when one eye has sustained significant damage and the IOP is high in the fellow eye despite maximum tolerable medical therapy (MTMT)—some surgeons will recommend surgery prior to unequivocal detection of damage.

Weinreb RN, Mills RP, eds. *Glaucoma Surgery: Principles and Techniques.* 2nd ed. Ophthalmology Monograph 4. San Francisco: American Academy of Ophthalmology; 1998:20.

The concept of MTMT merits discussion. The physician can determine that the patient is at maximum tolerable medical therapy only by advancing therapy beyond the tolerated level and documenting intolerance. This process can be frustrating for the physician and patient alike. An alternative concept is *core therapy,* in which treatment consists of those medications likely to work well in combination. If a patient does not have a satisfactory IOP response, a few alterations may be made, but it is likely that further medical intervention will simply delay indicated surgery.

Failure of medical therapy may be a result of noncompliance, which is a relative indication for surgery. Sometimes patients use their medications only around the time of an office visit. Thus, there may be progression despite apparent acceptable IOP. It is difficult to elicit an accurate history in this situation.

Although the hallmark of glaucoma is progressive optic nerve damage, it is actually relatively uncommon to make a surgical decision based on the detection of progressive change in the optic nerve or peripapillary retina. Progression of visual field damage is a far more common clinical indication for surgery, even though multiple field examinations may be required to determine with certainty that a damaged field has become more damaged. Many decisions to operate are based on a clinical judgment that the IOP is too high considering the stage of the disease. Thus, while an IOP of 25 mm Hg is not an indication for surgery in an eye with ocular hypertension, surgery may be indicated to lower this IOP in the setting of advanced glaucomatous optic neuropathy with only a small central field remaining. It is not always necessary to perform laser trabeculoplasty before proceeding to trabeculectomy. Certain conditions tend not to respond well to LTP. Eyes with very high IOP and advanced damage are unlikely to achieve substantial and sufficient IOP lowering with LTP.

***Contraindications***    Relative contraindications for glaucoma filtering surgery can be ocular or systemic. A blind eye should not be considered for incisional surgery. Ciliary body ablation is a better alternative for lowering IOP in such eyes if necessary for pain control, although even this procedure is not without risk. The risk of sympathetic ophthalmia should always be kept in mind when any procedure on a blind eye or an eye with poor visual potential is considered. Conditions that predispose to trabeculectomy failure such as active anterior segment neovascularization (rubeosis iridis) or active iritis are relative contraindications. The underlying problem should be addressed first, or a surgical alternative such as tube implant surgery (see below) should be considered. It may be extremely difficult to perform a successful trabeculectomy in an eye that has sustained extensive conjunctival injury or has an extremely thin sclera from extensive prior surgery or necrotizing scleritis. This is sometimes the case following trauma or retinal detachment surgery.

Filtering surgery is less successful in younger or aphakic/pseudophakic patients. A lower success rate is also found in patients with uveitic glaucoma or with previously failed filtration procedures. Black patients have a higher failure rate with filtering surgery.

***Preoperative evaluation***  The patient must be medically stable for an invasive ocular procedure under local anesthesia. Preoperative evaluation should determine and document factors that may affect surgical planning as well as those that determine the structural and functional status of the eye.

Control of preoperative inflammation with corticosteroids helps to reduce postoperative iritis and scarring of the filtering bleb. Anticholinesterase agents should be discontinued if possible and replaced temporarily by alternative medications at least 2–3 weeks before surgery to reduce bleeding and iridocyclitis.

In preparation for surgery, IOP should be reduced as close as possible to normal levels before surgery is performed, to minimize the risk of expulsive choroidal hemorrhage. Antiplatelet medications should be discontinued, and systemic hypertension should be controlled.

Patients should be informed of the purpose and expectations of surgery: to arrest or delay progressive visual loss caused by their glaucoma. They should understand that glaucoma surgery alone rarely improves vision and that glaucoma medications may still be required postoperatively, that surgery may fail completely, that vision could be lost as a result of surgery, and that glaucoma may progress despite successful surgery.

It is important to note that patients with far advanced visual field loss or field loss that is impinging on fixation are at risk for total loss of central acuity following a surgical procedure. The mechanism of this phenomenon is not known, but possibilities include

- Cystoid macular edema

- Early postoperative IOP spiking

- Shifting of the lamina, further compromising remaining axons

- Optic nerve ischemia, possibly related to regional anesthesia

> Costa VP, Smith M, Spaeth GL, et al. Loss of visual acuity after trabeculectomy. *Ophthalmology.* 1993;100:599–612.

***Trabeculectomy technique***  Knowledge of both the internal and external anatomy of the limbal area is essential for successful incisional surgery results. Trabeculectomy is a guarded partial-thickness filtering procedure performed by removing a block of limbal tissue beneath a scleral flap. The scleral flap provides resistance and limits the outflow of aqueous, thereby reducing the complications associated with early hypotony such as flat anterior chamber, cataract, serous and hemorrhagic choroidal effusion, macular edema, and optic nerve edema.

Because of the lower incidence of postoperative complications, trabeculectomy is the most commonly performed filtering operation. The use of antifibrotic agents such as mitomycin-C and 5-fluorouracil, combined with techniques of releasable sutures or laser suture lysis, enhances the longevity of guarded procedures, offers lower IOPs, and avoids some of the complications associated with full-thickness procedures.

Successful trabeculectomy surgery involves reducing IOP and avoiding or managing complications. Unlike cataract surgery, the success of trabeculectomy often depends on appropriate and timely postoperative intervention to influence the functioning of the filter. Complete healing of the epithelial and conjunctival wound with incomplete healing of the scleral wound is the goal of this procedure.

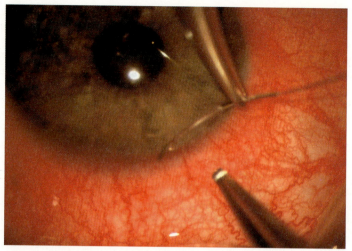

FIG VIII-2—Exposure for trabeculectomy: A corneal traction suture (shown) or superior rectus bridle suture (see Figure VIII-3) is inserted.

A trabeculectomy can be broken down into several basic steps:

□ *Preoperative evaluation:* As discussed above, before contemplating a surgical procedure, the ophthalmologist must consider factors such as the patient's general health, presumed life expectancy, and status of the fellow eye.

□ *Exposure:* A corneal traction suture or superior rectus bridle suture can rotate the globe down, giving excellent exposure of the superior sulcus and limbus, which can be very helpful for a limbus-based conjunctival flap (Fig VIII-2). The speculum should be adjusted to keep pressure off the globe.

□ *Conjunctival wound:* A fornix-based or limbus-based conjunctival flap can be used (Fig VIII-3). Each technique has advantages and disadvantages. The fornix-based flap provides better exposure at the limbus, and it is easier to do when a skilled assistant is not available. However, it is more difficult to achieve a water-tight closure with this incision. The limbus-based conjunctival flap is technically more challenging but allows for a secure closure well away from the limbus. The incision should be positioned 8–10 mm posterior to the limbus, and care should be taken to avoid the tendon of the superior rectus muscle. The conjunctival flap may be dissected either superiorly at 12:00 o'clock or in either superior quadrant, depending on surgeon preference.

□ *Scleral flap:* The exact size and shape of the scleral flap does not seem critical. Rather it is the relationship of the flap to the underlying sclerostomy that provides resistance to outflow. Although flap design will vary by surgeon preference, a common technique involves creating a 3–4 mm trapezoidal or rectangular flap (Fig VIII-4). It is important to dissect the flap anteriorly into clear cornea. The term trabeculectomy may have become a misnomer, as most surgeons prefer to remove a peripheral corneal block. When the flap is too far posterior, the risk of bleeding from iris root and ciliary body is greater.

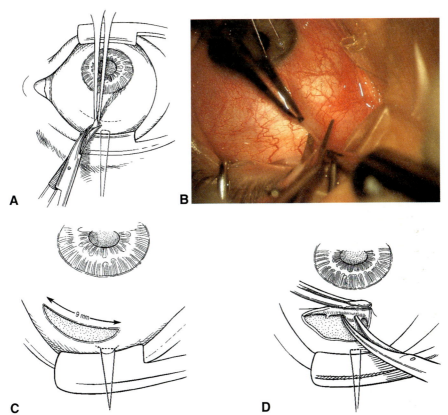

FIG VIII-3—Conjunctival flap is created. *A,* Drawing shows initial incision through conjunctiva and Tenon's capsule. *B,* Clinical photograph corresponding to *A* shows the initial incision for the creation of a limbus-based conjunctival flap. *C,* Completion of conjunctiva–Tenon's incision 8–9 mm posterior to limbus. *D,* Anterior dissection of conjunctiva–Tenon's flap with excision of Tenon's episcleral fibrous adhesions. (Illustrations reproduced with permission from Weinreb RN, Mills RP, eds. *Glaucoma Surgery: Principles and Techniques.* 2nd ed. Ophthalmology Monograph 4. San Francisco: American Academy of Ophthalmology; 1998:29–31.)

▫ *Paracentesis* (Fig VIII-5): To enable the surgeon to control the anterior chamber, a paracentesis should be performed. This procedure allows for gradual lowering of IOP, control of the anterior chamber through installation of basic saline solution (BSS) or viscoelastic, and intraoperative testing of the patency of the filtration site as well as of the integrity of the conjunctival closure. BSS is instilled through the paracentesis and sutures are added to the scleral flap until the flow is judged to be satisfactory. When a postoperative flat chamber occurs, the paracentesis already in place is used to re-form the chamber, which is much safer than trying to create a paracentesis in an eye with a flat chamber.

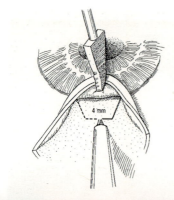

**A**

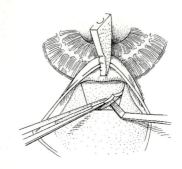

**B**

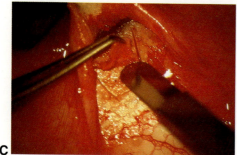

**C**

FIG VIII-4—Creation of the scleral flap. *A,* Preparation of split-thickness scleral flap 4 mm wide at base and 2.5 mm wide at apex. Flap is 2.5 mm in height. *B,* Dissection of scleral flap from scleral bed with spatula blade. (Illustrations reproduced with permission from Weinreb RN, Mills RP, eds. *Glaucoma Surgery: Principles and Techniques.* 2nd ed. Ophthalmology Monograph 4. San Francisco: American Academy of Ophthalmology; 1998:33.) *C,* Clinical photograph corresponding to *B* shows trapezoidal scleral flap.

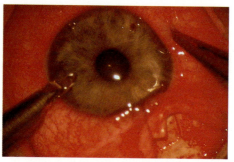

FIG VIII-5—Paracentesis is created through clear cornea.

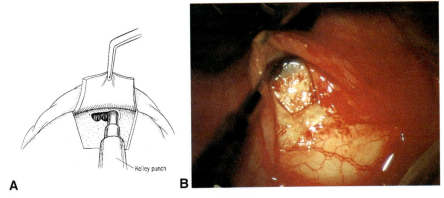

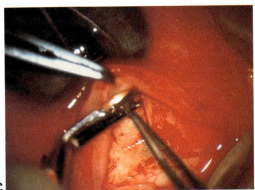

**A**

**B**

**C**

FIG VIII-6—Sclerostomy and iridectomy created with a punch or with sharp dissection. *A,* Schematic shows a sclerostomy created with a Kelley punch. (Illustration reproduced with permission from Weinreb RN, Mills RP, eds. *Glaucoma Surgery: Principles and Techniques.* 2nd ed. Ophthalmology Monograph 4. San Francisco: American Academy of Ophthalmology; 1998: 34.) *B,* Clinical photograph corresponds to *A. C,* Peripheral iridectomy is made with iridectomy scissors.

☐ *Sclerostomy:* The sclerostomy can be created with a punch or with sharp dissection (Fig VIII-6). The size of the ostomy is determined by the scleral flap and the amount of overlap desired by the surgeon. A small amount of tissue should remain at the edges of the ostomy to allow for resistance to outflow from the flap.

☐ *Iridectomy:* Most surgeons perform an iridectomy in order to lessen the risk of iris occluding the ostomy and to reduce the risk of pupillary block (see Figure VIII-6C). Care should be taken to avoid amputating ciliary processes or disrupting the zonular fibers or hyaloid face.

☐ *Closure of scleral flap:* With the advent of laser suture lysis and releasable sutures, many surgeons close the flap relatively tightly to avoid early shallow chambers. After a few days, flap sutures are released to promote filtration. Flow should be tested around the flap before closing the conjunctiva (Fig VIII-7). Leakage around the flap may be adjusted intraoperatively by the placement of additional sutures, removal of sutures, or application of cautery to shrink the wound edges.

☐ *Closure of conjunctiva:* Many techniques have been developed for conjunctival closure (Fig VIII-8). For a fornix-based flap, conjunctiva is secured at the limbus. For a limbus-based flap, conjunctiva and Tenon's capsule are closed separately or in a single layer.

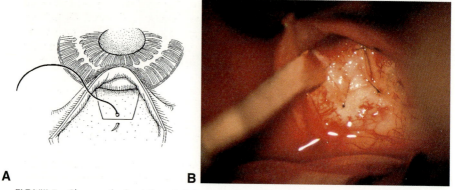

**A**  **B**

FIG VIII-7—Closure of scleral flap. *A,* Schematic illustration. (Illustration reproduced with permission from Weinreb RN, Mills RP, eds. *Glaucoma Surgery: Principles and Techniques.* 2nd ed. Ophthalmology Monograph 4. San Francisco: American Academy of Ophthalmology; 1998:36.) *B,* Flap closure is tested for flow with a surgical spear.

- □ *Postoperative management:* The success of glaucoma surgery depends on careful postoperative management. Topical antibiotics and corticosteroids are typically administered 4–6 times daily initially and tapered as the clinical course dictates. Cycloplegic agents (atropine) or mydriatics (phenylephrine) may also be used.

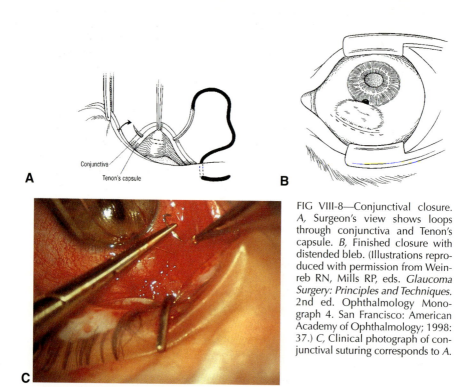

FIG VIII-8—Conjunctival closure. *A,* Surgeon's view shows loops through conjunctiva and Tenon's capsule. *B,* Finished closure with distended bleb. (Illustrations reproduced with permission from Weinreb RN, Mills RP, eds. *Glaucoma Surgery: Principles and Techniques.* 2nd ed. Ophthalmology Monograph 4. San Francisco: American Academy of Ophthalmology; 1998: 37.) *C,* Clinical photograph of conjunctival suturing corresponds to *A.*

***Antifibrotic agents***  The application of antifibrotic agents such as 5-fluorouracil (5-FU) and mitomycin-C (MMC) results in greater success and lower IOP following trabeculectomy. However, serious postoperative complications may occur, and these agents must not be used indiscriminantly. Antifibrotic agents should be used with caution in primary trabeculectomies on young myopic patients because of an increased risk of hypotony.

5-fluorouracil, a pyrimidine analogue, inhibits fibroblast proliferation and has proven useful in reducing scarring after filtering surgery. 5-fluorouracil undergoes intracellular conversion to the active deoxynucleotide 5-fluoro-2'-deoxyuridine 5'-monophosphate (FdUMP), which interferes with DNA synthesis through its action on thymidylate synthetase.

Although it was originally advocated for high-risk groups such as patients with aphakic/pseudophakic eyes, neovascular glaucoma, or a history of previous failed operations, this agent is now used on a routine basis by many surgeons. 5-FU (50 mg/ml on a surgical sponge) may be used intraoperatively in a fashion similar to that described below for mitomycin-C. Regimens for postoperative administration vary according to the observed healing response. A total of 5 mg in 0.1–0.5 cc can be injected with relatively mild discomfort. The total dose can be titrated to the observed healing response and corneal toxicity. Complications such as corneal epithelial defects commonly occur and require discontinuation of 5-FU injections. The site of injection can be varied from 180° away to adjacent to the bleb.

Mitomycin-C is a naturally occurring antibiotic-antineoplastic compound that is derived from *Streptomyces caespitosus*. It acts as an alkylating agent after enzyme activation resulting in DNA cross-linking. Mitomycin-C is a potent antifibrotic agent. It is most commonly administered intraoperatively by placing a surgical sponge soaked in MMC within the subconjunctival space in contact with sclera at the planned trabeculectomy site. Concentrations in current usage are typically between 0.2 and 0.4 mg/ml with a duration of application from 1 to 4 minutes. Little data are available to compare regimens, and most surgeons will increase concentration or duration based on risk factors for trabeculectomy failure.

***Flap closure***  Techniques allowing tighter initial wound closure of the scleral flap help to prevent early postoperative hypotony. The use of releasable flap sutures or the placement of additional sutures that can be cut postoperatively to facilitate outflow following trabeculectomy are two of these techniques. In laser suture lysis the conjunctiva is compressed with either a Zeiss goniolens or a lens designed for suture lysis (Hoskins, Ritch, Mandelkorn), and the argon laser (set at 300–400 mW, 100 µm, and 0.02–0.1 second) can usually lyse the selected nylon suture with one application. It is important to avoid creating a full-thickness conjunctival burn. Shorter duration of laser energy and avoidance of pigment or blood are helpful. Krypton laser may allow suture lysis in patients with subconjunctival hemorrhage. Most surgeons wait at least 48 hours before performing laser suture lysis. Filtration is best enhanced if lysis or suture release is completed within 2 weeks or before the flap has fibrosed. This period is lengthened to several months when antifibrotic agents have been used.

***Postoperative considerations in filtering surgery***  Topical cycloplegic agents, antibiotics, and corticosteroids are administered postoperatively. Sub-Tenon's corticosteroids or a short course of systemic corticosteroids may be administered to reduce scarring and inflammation, especially in patients with poor prognoses. When the postoperative course is uneventful, steroids are slowly tapered. Unfortunately, the

TABLE VIII-1

COMPLICATIONS OF FILTERING SURGERY

| EARLY COMPLICATIONS | LATE COMPLICATIONS |
| --- | --- |
| Infection | Leakage or failure of the filtering bleb |
| Hypotony | Cataract |
| Flat anterior chamber | Blebitis |
| Aqueous misdirection | Endophthalmitis/bleb infection |
| Hyphema | Symptomatic bleb (dysesthetic bleb) |
| Formation or acceleration of cataract | Bleb migration |
| Transient IOP elevation | Hypotony |
| Cystoid macular edema | |
| Hypotony maculopathy | |
| Choroidal effusion | |
| Suprachoroidal hemorrhage | |
| Persistent uveitis | |
| Dellen formation | |
| Loss of vision | |

postoperative course is rarely uneventful, and much of the care is aimed at preventing or managing complications.

***Complications of filtering surgery***   Early and late complications of filtering surgery are listed in Table VIII-1. The filtering bleb can leak, produce dellen, or expand so as to interfere with eyelid function or extend onto the cornea and interfere with vision or cause irritation. Filtering blebs are dynamic. They evolve over time and must be monitored. All patients must be informed of the warning signs of endophthalmitis and instructed to seek ophthalmic care immediately should any signs develop.

The techniques of choroidal tap and anterior chamber re-formation should be familiar to any surgeon who performs filtering surgery, which incurs the risk of flat chamber associated with choroidal detachment. Suprachoroidal fluid is drained through one or more posterior sclerotomies, as the chamber is deepened through a paracentesis.

The use of contact lenses with a filtering bleb presents special problems. Contact lenses may be difficult to fit in the presence of a filtering bleb, or the lens may ride against the bleb, causing discomfort and increasing the risk of infection. Several options can be considered for the high myope needing trabeculectomy who prefers not to wear spectacles:

◻ PRK or LASIK prior to trabeculectomy

◻ Intracorneal ring segments

◻ Clear lens extraction before or after trabeculectomy

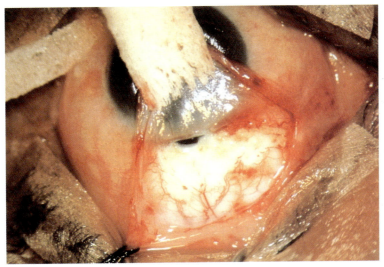

FIG VIII-9—Intraoperative photograph of full-thickness sclerectomy performed with Descemet's punch.

When an initial filtering procedure is not adequate to control the glaucoma and resumption of medical therapy is not successful, revision of original surgery, repeat filtering surgery at a new site, or tube-shunt and possibly cyclodestructive procedures may be indicated.

Camras CB. Diagnosis and management of complications of glaucoma filtering surgery. In: *Focal Points: Clinical Modules for Ophthalmologists.* San Francisco: American Academy of Ophthalmology; 1994: vol 12, no 3.

Haynes WL, Alward WL. Control of intraocular pressure after trabeculectomy. *Surv Ophthalmol.* 1999;43:345–355.

## Full-Thickness Sclerectomy

Full-thickness filtering operations are performed by removing a block of limbal tissue with a punch, trephine, laser, or cautery (Fig VIII-9). The advantage of full-thickness filtering procedures is that they lower IOP and can maintain the lowered level for long periods of time. Historically, ophthalmic surgeons performed these procedures on patients in whom a postoperative IOP lowered to the mid to high teens would not be considered adequate. Currently, the use of concurrent or subsequent antifibrotic agents such as MMC or 5-FU may equalize the IOP outcomes for full-thickness and guarded filtering procedures. The disadvantages of full-thickness compared with partial-thickness techniques include a higher incidence of postoperative flat anterior chamber, cataract, hypotony, choroidal effusion, leakage of filtering blebs, and endophthalmitis.

## Combined Cataract and Filtering Surgery

Both cataract and glaucoma are conditions that show increasing prevalence with aging. It is not surprising that many patients with glaucoma eventually develop cataracts either naturally or as a result of the effects of glaucoma therapy.

*Indications*   Indications for combining glaucoma surgery (usually trabeculectomy) with cataract extraction include the following:

- □ Glaucoma that is uncontrollable either medically or after laser trabeculoplasty when visual function is significantly impaired by a cataract
- □ Cataract requiring extraction in a glaucoma patient who has advanced visual field loss
- □ Cataract requiring extraction in a glaucoma patient requiring medications to control IOP in whom medical therapy is poorly tolerated
- □ Cataract requiring extraction in a glaucoma patient who requires multiple medications to control IOP

*Contraindications*   Combined cataract and filtering surgery should be avoided in the following situations, in which glaucoma surgery alone is preferred:

- □ Glaucoma that requires a very low target IOP
- □ Advanced glaucoma with uncontrolled IOP and immediate need for successful reduction of IOP

*Considerations*   A combined procedure may prevent a postoperative rise in IOP. Combined procedures are generally less effective than filtering procedures alone in controlling IOP over time, although combined procedures using small-incision phacoemulsification techniques with an antifibrotic agent appear to have improved success rates that more closely mirror those of trabeculectomy alone. For patients in whom glaucoma is the greatest immediate threat to vision, filtering surgery alone may be performed first. The postoperative discontinuation of miotics, if used, is often enough to increase visual acuity so that cataract extraction and IOL implantation may be delayed.

Several clinical challenges are common in patients with coexisting cataract and glaucoma. Medical therapy for glaucoma may create chronic miosis, and the surgeon must deal with a small pupil. Patients with exfoliation syndrome often have fragile zonular support of the lens, and vitreous loss is therefore more common in such complicated eyes. As with all surgery, the risks, benefits, and alternatives should be discussed with the patient.

*Technique*   Several surgical approaches to coexisting cataract and glaucoma are now in use, and a debate has surfaced with the development of successful small-incision clear corneal cataract extraction. Single-site combined surgery with phacoemulsification had been the commonly accepted approach when a scleral tunnel technique was used. Two-site surgery with a clear corneal cataract extraction and a standard trabeculectomy has recently gained in popularity. For patients who have IOP controlled medically, clear corneal cataract surgery alone may be the appropriate choice. As no violation of conjunctiva or sclera occurs, there is little reason to perform an incidental trabeculectomy. Rather, standard trabeculectomy can be performed when dictated by independent indications. Although little evidence exists to compare long-term outcomes with these different approaches, it makes sense for the surgeon to perform his or her best cataract procedure, as the primary indication for surgery is the presence of cataract.

Balyeat HD. Cataract surgery in the glaucoma patient. Part 1: A cataract surgeon's perspective. In: *Focal Points: Clinical Modules for Ophthalmologists.* San Francisco: American Academy of Ophthalmology; 1998: vol 16, no 3.

Skuta GL. Cataract surgery in the glaucoma patient. Part 2: A glaucoma surgeon's perspective. In: *Focal Points: Clinical Modules for Ophthalmologists.* San Francisco: American Academy of Ophthalmology; 1998: vol 16, no 4.

Weinreb RN, Mills RP, eds. *Glaucoma Surgery: Principles and Techniques.* 2nd ed. Ophthalmology Monograph 4. San Francisco: American Academy of Ophthalmology; 1998:65–85.

## Surgery for Angle-Closure Glaucoma

The first clinical decision point following the diagnosis of angle-closure glaucoma is to distinguish between angle closure based on a pupillary-block mechanism and angle closure based on another mechanism. Laser iridectomy is the procedure of choice to relieve pupillary block, but this is of no use in an eye with complete synechial closure as a result of neovascularization or chronic inflammation. It is sometimes necessary, however, to perform the iridectomy as much for diagnostic purposes as for therapeutic ones. For example, the diagnosis of plateau iris can be definitely confirmed only when a patent iridectomy fails to change peripheral iris configuration and relieve angle closure.

The treatment of pupillary-block glaucoma, whether primary or secondary, is a laser or an incisional iridectomy. These procedures provide an alternative route for aqueous trapped in the posterior chamber to enter the anterior chamber, allowing the iris to recede from its occlusion of the trabecular meshwork (Fig VIII-10). Laser surgery has become the preferred method in almost all cases. Both the argon laser and Nd:YAG laser are effective in relieving pupillary block. Following the successful resolution of pupillary block, IOP may return to normal or may remain elevated. At this point the indications for surgery become similar to those for POAG.

For eyes with secondary angle closure not caused by pupillary block, an attempt should be made to identify and treat underlying conditions. For example, an eye with rubeosis iridis from diabetic retinopathy should have retinal ablation prior to glaucoma surgery. In early cases the IOP elevation may be reversible. Even in the presence of complete synechial angle closure from rubeosis, the neovascularization may regress following retinal ablation, allowing subsequent successful trabeculectomy.

### Laser Iridectomy

**Indications**   The indications for iridectomy include the presence of pupillary block and the need to determine the presence of pupillary block. Laser iridectomy is also indicated to prevent pupillary block in an eye considered at risk, as determined by gonioscopic evaluation or because of an angle-closure attack in the fellow eye.

**Contraindications**   An eye with active rubeosis iridis may bleed following laser iridectomy. The risk of bleeding is also increased in a patient taking systemic anticoagulants, including aspirin. The argon laser may be more appropriate than the

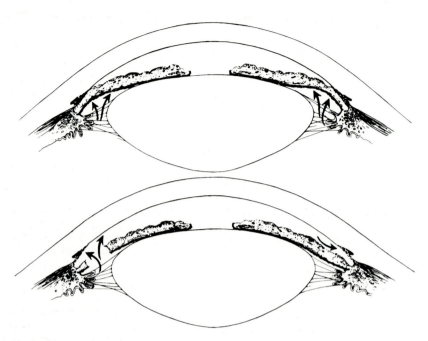

FIG VIII-10—Angle-closure glaucoma. Laser or surgical iridectomy breaks the pupillary block and results in opening of the entire peripheral angle if no permanent peripheral anterior synechiae are present. (Reproduced and modified with permission from Kolker AE, Hetherington J, eds. *Becker-Shaffer's Diagnosis and Therapy of the Glaucomas.* 5th ed. St Louis: Mosby; 1983.)

Nd:YAG should laser iridectomy be performed in such an individual. Although laser iridectomy is not helpful for angle closure not caused by a pupillary block mechanism, it is sometimes necessary to perform the laser iridectomy to ensure that pupillary block is not present.

***Preoperative consideration***    In the setting of acute angle closure it is often difficult to perform laser iridectomy because of the cloudy cornea, shallow chamber, and engorged iris. The clinician should attempt to break the attack medically, then proceed to surgery. It is easiest to penetrate the iris in a crypt. Care should be taken to keep the iridectomy peripheral and covered by eyelid, if possible, to avoid monocular diplopia. Pretreatment with pilocarpine may be helpful by stretching and thinning the iris. Pretreatment of IOP with apraclonidine or other agents can help blunt IOP spikes.

***Technique***    The argon laser may be used to produce an iridectomy in most eyes, but very dark and very light irides present technical difficulties. Using a condensing contact lens, the typical initial laser settings are 0.02–0.1 second of duration, 50-μm spot size, and 800–1000 mW of power. There are a number of variations in technique, and iris color dictates which technique is chosen. Complications include localized lens opacity, acute rise in IOP (which may damage the optic nerve), transient or persistent iritis, early closure of the iridectomy, and corneal and retinal burns.

The Q-switched Nd:YAG laser generally requires fewer pulses and less energy than an argon laser to create a patent iridectomy and has become the preferred technique for most eyes. Also, the effectiveness of this laser is not affected by iris color. With a condensing contact lens, the typical initial laser setting is 2–8 mJ. Potential complications include corneal burns, disruption of the anterior lens capsule or corneal endothelium, bleeding (usually transient), postoperative IOP spike, inflammation, and delayed closure of the iridectomy. To prevent damage to the lens the surgeon must use caution with the Q-switched Nd:YAG laser in performing further enlargement of the opening once patency is established. The location should be as peripheral as possible, where the distance between the iris and lens is greater.

***Postoperative care*** Bleeding may occur from the iridectomy site, particularly with Nd:YAG laser. Often, compression of the eye with the laser lens will tamponade the vessel. In rare cases when this does not work, it may be helpful to use the argon laser to coagulate the vessel. Postoperative pressure spikes may occur, as with LTP, and they are treated as described in the section on LTP. Inflammation is treated as necessary with topical corticosteroids.

***Complications*** The complications associated with a particular laser mode have been listed above in discussion of that laser. Potential complications from laser iridectomy in general include focal lens damage, retinal detachment, bleeding, and IOP spike. Lens damage can be avoided by ceasing the procedure as soon as the iris is penetrated. Retinal detachment is very rare but has been associated with Nd:YAG laser iridectomy. Bleeding and IOP spikes are discussed above.

Ritch R, Shields MB, Krupin T, eds. *The Glaucomas.* 2nd ed. St Louis: Mosby; 1996.

Shields MB. *Textbook of Glaucoma.* 4th ed. Baltimore: Williams & Wilkins; 1997: 490–496.

## Laser Gonioplasty or Peripheral Iridoplasty

***Indications*** Gonioplasty, or iridoplasty, is a technique to deepen the angle that is occasionally useful in angle-closure glaucoma resulting from plateau iris. Stromal burns are created with the argon laser in the peripheral iris to cause contraction and flattening. It is difficult to diagnose plateau iris unless an iridectomy has been created and the angle configuration has not changed and, therefore, remains occludable.

***Contraindications*** The contraindications are the same as those for laser iridectomy.

***Preoperative considerations*** An angle that is closed from plateau iris will not open with creation of a laser iridectomy, as the underlying mechanism is not pupillary block. This is often a difficult condition to diagnose accurately.

***Technique*** Typical laser settings are 0.1–0.5 second duration, 200–500 μm spot size, and 200–500 mW of power. This procedure can be used to open the angle temporarily, in anticipation of a more definitive laser or incisional iridectomy, or in other types of angle closure such as plateau iris syndrome and nanophthalmos.

## Incisional Surgery for Angle Closure

**Peripheral iridectomy**  Incisional surgical iridectomy may be required if a patent iridectomy cannot be achieved with a laser. Such situations include a cloudy cornea, a flat anterior chamber, and insufficient patient cooperation.

**Cataract extraction**  When pupillary block is associated with a visually significant cataract, lens extraction might be considered as a primary procedure. However, laser iridectomy may stop an acute attack of pupillary block, so that cataract surgery may be performed more safely at a later time.

**Chamber deepening and goniosynechialysis**  When PAS develop in cases of angle-closure glaucoma, iridectomy alone may not relieve the glaucoma adequately. Chamber deepening through a paracentesis with intraoperative gonioscopy may break PAS of relatively recent onset. A viscoelastic agent and/or cyclodialysis spatula may be useful, in a procedure known as *goniosynechialysis*, to break synechiae.

> Campbell DG, Vela A. Modern goniosynechialysis for the treatment of synechial angle-closure glaucoma. *Ophthalmology.* 1984;91:1052–1060.

## Other Procedures to Lower IOP

Incisional and nonincisional procedures to control IOP include tube-shunt surgery, ciliary body ablation, cyclodialysis, and viscocanalostomy and other nonpenetrating procedures.

### Glaucoma Tube Shunt

Many different types of devices have been developed that aid filtration by shunting aqueous to a site posterior to the limbus (Table VIII-2). The shunts, or drainage devices, in current use generally have a tube placed in the anterior chamber or through the pars plana that flows to an extraocular reservoir, which is placed in the equatorial region on the sclera (Fig VIII-11). They can be broadly categorized as resistance (valved) devices, also known as *flow-restricted,* or nonresistance (nonvalved) devices. The most popular nonresistance devices are the Molteno and Baerveldt designs. Popular resistance devices include the Krupin and Ahmed. The anterior chamber tube shunt to an encircling band (ACTSEB) described by Schocket used an

TABLE VIII-2

GLAUCOMA DRAINAGE DEVICES

| | BAERVELDT | | MOLTENO | | | |
| | 250 | 350 | SINGLE PLATE | DOUBLE PLATE | KRUPIN | AHMED |
|---|---|---|---|---|---|---|
| Surface area | 250 mm$^2$ | 350 mm$^2$ | 135 mm$^2$ | 270 mm$^2$ | 194 mm$^2$ | 184 mm$^2$ |
| Height profile | 0.84 mm | 0.84 mm | 2.16 mm | 2.16 mm | 2.54 mm | 1.90 mm |
| Plate material | Silicone | Silicone | Polypropylene | Polypropylene | Silicone | Polypropylene |
| Tube | Open | Open | Open | Open | Valve | Valve |

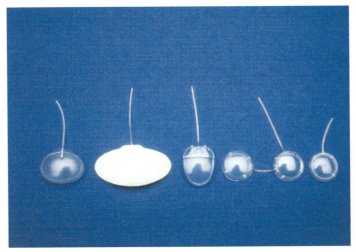

FIG VIII-11—Glaucoma drainage devices, from left to right: Krupin, Baerveldt, Ahmed, double-plate Molteno, single-plate Molteno.

encircling element intended for scleral buckling with tubing attached to the encircling band. A variation on the ACTSEB can be used on eyes with a scleral buckle.

Schocket SS, Nirankari VS, Lakhanpal V, et al. Anterior chamber tube shunt to an encircling band in the treatment of neovascular glaucoma and other refractory glaucomas: a long-term study. *Ophthalmology.* 1985;92:553–562.

Spiegel D, Shrader RR, Wilson RP. Anterior chamber tube shunt to an encircling band (Schocket procedure) in the treatment of refractory glaucoma. *Ophthalmic Surg.* 1992; 23:804–807.

**Indications**   The devices mentioned and other similar types of implants are generally reserved for difficult glaucoma cases in which conventional filtering surgery has failed or is likely to fail. One form of "failure" may be the inability of the patient to be a suitable candidate for trabeculectomy. The following clinical settings are some in which glaucoma tube shunt should be considered:

- *Trabeculectomy failure:* Failure of a trabeculectomy may lead to the need for further surgical intervention if IOP cannot be controlled medically.

- *Failed trabeculectomy with antifibrotics:* It may be appropriate to perform a repeat trabeculectomy in some clinical situations. However, when the factors that precipitated the initial failure cannot be modified, or when it is not technically possible to repeat the trabeculectomy, a glaucoma tube shunt may be the procedure of choice.

- *Active uveitis:* Although little randomized prospective data is available to compare trabeculectomy with antifibrotics to glaucoma tube shunt in the setting of active uveitis, the success of trabeculectomy in the setting of active inflammation is disappointingly low.

❑ *Neovascular glaucoma:* Eyes with neovascular glaucoma (NVG) are high risk for failure of a trabeculectomy. In one prospective study the 5-year success rate for trabeculectomy with 5-FU in NVG was 28%. When possible, retinal ablation is performed prior to glaucoma surgery in cases of NVG. When the IOP mandates urgent surgery, or when the NVG does not respond to retinal ablation, a glaucoma tube shunt is indicated.

❑ *Inadequate conjunctiva:* Following severe trauma or extensive surgery (e.g., retinal detachment surgery), conjunctiva is often inadequate or has too much scarring for trabeculectomy to be successful. A glaucoma tube shunt can be placed, even in the presence of a scleral buckle. When vitrectomy has been performed, the tube can be placed through the pars plana.

❑ *Impending need for penetrating keratoplasty (PK):* In an eye with elevated IOP requiring surgical lowering and corneal disease requiring PK, a glaucoma tube shunt may provide better long-term IOP control than repeat trabeculectomy.

Other factors should be considered when evaluating a patient for possible tube-shunt surgery:

❑ *Poor candidate for trabeculectomy:* In addition to the clinical settings described above, lack of an intact blood–aqueous barrier is a relative indication for a glaucoma tube shunt.

❑ *Potential for visual acuity:* It may not be appropriate to perform incisional surgery with a prolonged convalescence in an eye with little potential for useful vision. However, when the potential for useful vision remains, it is worth the risks and potentially complicated postoperative course of glaucoma tube-shunt surgery.

❑ *Need for lower IOP:* After a failed trabeculectomy, medical therapy should be resumed. If IOP is not controlled, additional surgery must be considered.

**Contraindications**   Tube-shunt surgery may have a complicated postoperative course. Thus, it is relatively contraindicated in eyes with very poor visual potential or for patients unable to comply with self-care in the postoperative period. Borderline corneal endothelial function is a relative contraindication for anterior chamber placement of a tube.

**Preoperative considerations**   Preoperative evaluation should be similar to that for trabeculectomy. During the ophthalmic examination, the clinician should note the status of the conjunctiva, the health of the sclera at the anticipated tube and external reservoir sites, and the location of vitreous in the eye.

**Techniques**   Although devices differ in design, the basic techniques for implantation are similar. The superotemporal quadrant is preferred, as surgical access is more easily achieved than in the superonasal quadrant. The extraocular plate or valve mechanism is sutured between the vertical and horizontal rectus muscles posterior to the muscle insertions. The tube is then routed anteriorly to enter in the chamber angle or through the pars plana for posterior implantation in eyes that have had a vitrectomy. Typically, the tube is covered with tissue such as sclera, pericardium, or dura to help prevent erosion.

For the nonresistance devices there are a number of techniques to restrict flow in the early postoperative period, such as putting a suture in the lumen of the tube or ligating the tube. This is not necessary with the resistance devices, but hypotony and a flat chamber can still occur despite the presence of a valve. It is not clear at present whether antifibrotic agents improve the success of glaucoma tube-shunt surgery. For those devices with two plates the second plate and its interconnecting tube may be placed either over or under the superior rectus muscle, and the distal plate is attached to the sclera in a manner similar to the proximal plate.

**Postoperative management**    The IOP in the early postoperative period can be high, low, or in between. Early IOP spikes are best managed medically. After sufficient time has passed for a capsule to form around the extraocular reservoir, the occluding suture is released for the nonresistance devices. Topical corticosteroids, antibiotics, and cycloplegics are used as with trabeculectomy. An IOP spike is expected around 2–8 weeks postoperatively, which probably represents encapsulation around the extraocular reservoir. Aqueous suppression can control the IOP, and this elevation usually resolves spontaneously within 1–6 months.

**Complications**    Success rates have been encouraging, but the implant procedures share many of the complications associated with conventional filtering surgery. Unique problems related to the tubes and plates also arise. Early overfiltration in an eye with the tube in the anterior chamber results in a flat chamber and tube–cornea touch. This can compromise the cornea. Even when no touch occurs, an area of corneal decompensation can appear near the tube. Tube migration in the eye or tube erosion may require surgical revision. Eyes must be monitored for late complications such as tube erosion or migration. Table VIII-3 lists several common complications with methods to avoid or manage them.

### Ciliary Body Ablation Procedures

Several surgical procedures reduce aqueous secretion by destroying a portion of the ciliary body. The secretory activity of ciliary body epithelium can be inhibited by treatment with cyclocryotherapy; diathermy; therapeutic ultrasound; and thermal lasers such as continuous-wave Nd:YAG, argon, and diode.

**Indications**    Ciliary ablation is indicated to lower IOP in eyes that have poor visual potential or are poor candidates for incisional surgery. Surgery for blind eyes should be avoided, if possible, because of the small risk of sympathetic ophthalmia. Interventions such as retrobulbar alcohol injection or enucleation can be considered for blind painful eyes. Ciliary body ablation is generally reserved for eyes that have been or are likely to be unresponsive to other modes of therapy.

**Contraindications**    Ciliary ablation is relatively contraindicated in eyes with good vision because of the risk of loss of visual acuity.

**Preoperative evaluation**    This step is the same as for incisional glaucoma surgery.

**Methods and considerations**    *Cyclocryotherapy* has been the most commonly used of these methods over the past few decades. However, interest has been increasing in *transscleral Nd:YAG* and *transscleral diode laser cyclophotocoagulation,* both of which appear to cause less pain and inflammation than cyclocryotherapy. An *endoscopic laser delivery system* has been advocated for use combined with cataract

TABLE VIII-3

COMPLICATIONS OF GLAUCOMA TUBE-SHUNT SURGERY
AND PREVENTION/MANAGEMENT OPTIONS

| COMPLICATION | PREVENTION/MANAGEMENT |
|---|---|
| Tube–cornea touch | Avoid by making the anterior chamber insertion parallel with the iris plane and using a tube occlusion technique to avoid a flat chamber. Pars plana insertion avoids this complication. |
| Flat chamber and hypotony | Flat chamber and hypotony caused by overfiltration are best avoided by using a resistance device, an occlusion technique, or viscoelastic agents. A flat chamber with tube–cornea touch and serous choroidal detachment should be managed by early drainage of choroidal effusion and re-formation of the anterior chamber. Viscoelastic can help maintain the chamber. A flat chamber resulting from a complication such as suprachoroid-al hemorrhage must be managed based on the clinical setting. |
| Tube occlusion | Avoid by positioning tube away from uveal tissue (iris) or vitreous. A generous vitrectomy should be performed if needed. Although it is possible to use Nd:YAG laser to clear an occlusion, surgical intervention is often required. |
| Tube migration | Avoid by meticulous tube placement and coverage. Different materials used to cover the tube may vary in rate of degradation. It may be possible to reposition a tube with extraocular manipulation only. A new entry site can be fashioned without disturbing the capsule around the extraocular plate. Some surgeons suture the tube to the sclera with an S-curve in an effort to prevent extraocular scarring from causing tube migration. |
| Valve malfunction | Valves should be tested for patency prior to insertion of the tube. Several techniques have been described to unclog a valve. |
| Tube or plate exposure or erosion | Conjunctiva must not be under tension when covering the tube or plate. Most surgeons use a patch graft such as sclera or pericardium to cover the tube. Exposure increases the risk of endophthalmitis. In some settings the device should be removed if adequate coverage cannot be achieved. |

surgery or in pseudophakic and aphakic eyes. Use of the argon laser aimed at the ciliary processes through a goniolens is possible in a small percentage of patients.

**Postoperative management**   Pain following these procedures may be substantial, and patients should be provided with adequate analgesics, including narcotics, during the immediate postoperative period.

**Complications**   Each of these procedures may result in prolonged hypotony, pain, inflammation, cystoid macular edema, hemorrhage, and even phthisis bulbi. Sympathetic ophthalmia is a rare but serious complication.

## Cyclodialysis

Cyclodialysis creates a direct communication between the anterior chamber and the suprachoroidal space. It can occur traumatically or surgically.

**Indications**   Cyclodialysis is rarely performed, but it may be helpful in aphakic patients who have not responded to filtering surgery.

**Technique**   A small scleral incision is made approximately 4 mm from the limbus, and a fine spatula is passed under the sclera into the anterior chamber. This spatula disinserts a portion of the ciliary muscle from the scleral spur and creates a cleft in the angle, providing direct communication between the anterior chamber and the suprachoroidal space.

**Complications**   Bleeding, inflammation, cataract, and the stripping of Descemet's membrane are possible complications. Profound hypotony, or an equally significant rise in IOP should the cleft close, may also occur. Some surgeons have advocated cyclodialysis combined with cataract surgery for patients with glaucoma, but this approach is not widely accepted.

## Nonpenetrating Procedures (Viscocanalostomy)

Although the most widely accepted IOP-lowering incisional surgeries involve creating a direct communication between the anterior chamber and the subconjunctival space, nonpenetrating surgery has also been proposed. Zimmerman and colleagues first described the nonpenetrating trabeculectomy in the early 1980s. The goal was to achieve IOP lowering while avoiding some of the complications of standard trabeculectomy.

Recently, interest in nonpenetrating surgery has been revived. Several variations all involve a deep sclerectomy. These include deep sclerectomy with collagen implant, and deep sclerectomy with injection of viscoelastic into Schlemm's canal (viscocanalostomy). These techniques involve creation of a superficial scleral flap and a deeper scleral dissection underneath to leave behind only a thin layer of sclera and Descemet's membrane.

At present, there is little long-term prospective randomized data comparing these new procedures with trabeculectomy. In theory, nonpenetrating surgery may avoid some of the complications associated with penetrating filtering surgery. However, the procedures are technically challenging, and preliminary results suggest that IOP reduction may be less than with trabeculectomy.

## Congenital/Infantile Glaucoma

Terminology surrounding the glaucomas of childhood is often imprecise (see also chapter VI). For those glaucomas occurring within the first few years of life, surgery is the appropriate treatment. Trabeculotomy and goniotomy are the preferred procedures in congenital/infantile glaucoma. Goniotomy is possible only in an eye with a relatively clear cornea, whereas trabeculotomy can be performed whether the cornea is clear or cloudy. A standard trabeculotomy performed superiorly can be converted to trabeculectomy if needed. Published success rates are similar for trabeculotomy and goniotomy.

For an eye that has failed one of these procedures, debate continues whether the next procedure should be trabeculectomy with an antifibrotic agent, glaucoma drainage device, or ciliary ablation. These procedures in infants are probably best performed by those clinicians experienced in the surgical treatment of childhood glaucomas. BCSC Section 6, *Pediatric Ophthalmology and Strabismus,* discusses these issues in chapter XXI, Pediatric Glaucomas.

## Goniotomy and Trabeculotomy

**Indications**   The presence of childhood glaucoma is an indication for surgery. The selection of procedure will, in part, depend on the training and experience of the surgeon.

**Contraindications**   Contraindications to surgery include an infant with unstable health, an infant with multiple anomalies with poor prognosis, and a grossly disorganized eye.

**Preoperative evaluation**   Thorough examination in the office is not always possible. Sometimes a bottle feeding will distract a young infant enough to allow tonometry and dilated examination. When this is not possible, examination under anesthesia is necessary. Surgery can be performed at the same or at a subsequent session. It is best not to dilate the eye expected to have angle surgery in order to better protect the lens during the procedure. BCSC Section 6 includes a chapter on examination techniques and tips written by pediatric ophthalmologists.

**Technique**   The anterior chamber should be filled with viscoelastic to prevent collapse and to tamponade bleeding. With a *goniotomy* a needle-knife is passed across the anterior chamber, and a superficial incision is made in the anterior aspect of the trabecular meshwork under gonioscopic control (Fig VIII-12). A clear cornea is necessary to provide an adequate view of the chamber angle.

In a *trabeculotomy* a fine wirelike instrument (trabeculotome) is inserted into Schlemm's canal from an external incision, and the trabecular meshwork is torn by rotating the trabeculotome into the anterior chamber (Fig VIII-13, p 174). Schlemm's canal is more easily identified if a partial-thickness scleral flap is first elevated, similar to trabeculectomy. A gradual cutdown can then be made in order to better identify the canal. Alternative techniques have been developed in which a prolene or nylon suture is threaded through Schlemm's canal and the end is retrieved. The two ends of the suture are then pulled and the suture ruptures the trabecular meshwork and passes into the anterior chamber. The suture is then removed. This process may be performed over 180° or 360° of the angle. Trabeculotomy is particularly useful if the cornea is too cloudy to allow adequate visualization for goniotomy. However, the abnormal angle anatomy associated with congenital glaucomas sometimes precludes localization of Schlemm's canal.

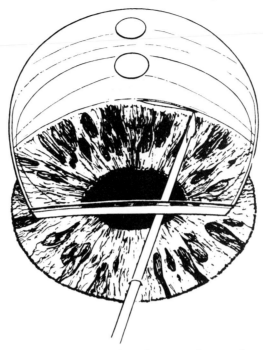

FIG VIII-12—Goniotomy incision as seen through a surgical contact lens. (Reproduced with permission from Shaffer RN. *Am J Ophthalmol.* 1966;62:613-618. Copyright by the Ophthalmic Publishing Company.)

***Complications*** Complications of both of these operations include hyphema, infection, lens damage, and uveitis. Descemet's membrane may be stripped during trabeculotomy. General anesthesia may cause serious complications in children, and bilateral procedures are indicated in some children because of anesthetic risks. There is a long-term risk of amblyopia, and the child must be followed closely over time. IOP elevation may recur at any time.

Beck AD, Lynch MG. Pediatric glaucoma. In: *Focal Points Clinical Modules for Ophthalmologists.* San Francisco: American Academy of Ophthalmology. 1997: vol 15, no 5.

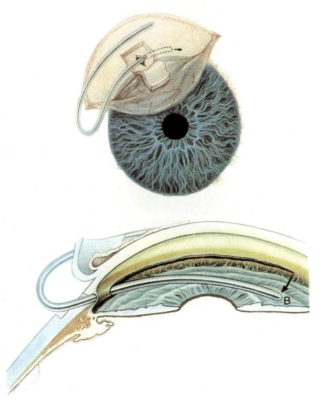

FIG VIII-13—Trabeculotomy. *Top,* Probe is gently passed along Schlemm's canal with little resistance for 6–10 mm. *Bottom,* By rotating the probe internally (B), the surgeon ruptures the trabeculum, and the probe appears in the anterior chamber with minimum bleeding. (Reproduced and modified with permission from Kolker AE, Hetherington J, eds. *Becker-Shaffer's Diagnosis and Therapy of the Glaucomas.* 5th ed. St Louis: Mosby; 1983.)

# BASIC TEXTS

## Glaucoma

Anderson DR, Patella VM. *Automated Static Perimetry*. 2nd ed. St Louis: Mosby; 1999.

Drance SM, Anderson DR, eds. *Automatic Perimetry in Glaucoma: A Practical Guide*. Orlando, FL: Grune & Stratton; 1985.

Epstein DL, Allingham RR, Schuman JS, eds. *Chandler and Grant's Glaucoma*. 4th ed. Baltimore: Williams & Willkins; 1997.

Harrington DO, Drake MV. *The Visual Fields: A Textbook and Atlas of Clinical Perimetry*. 6th ed. St Louis: Mosby; 1989.

Hart WM Jr, ed. *Adler's Physiology of the Eye: Clinical Application*. 9th ed. St Louis: Mosby; 1992.

Minckler DS, Van Buskirk EM, eds. Glaucoma. In: Wright KW, ed. *Color Atlas of Ophthalmic Surgery*. Philadelphia: Lippincott; 1992.

Ritch R, Shields MB, Krupin T, eds. *The Glaucomas*. 2nd ed. St Louis: Mosby; 1996.

Shields MB. *Textbook of Glaucoma*. 4th ed. Baltimore: Williams & Wilkins; 1997.

Stamper RL, Lieberman MF, Drake MV, eds. *Becker-Shaffer's Diagnosis and Therapy of the Glaucomas*. 7th ed. St Louis: Mosby; 1999.

Tasman W, Jaeger EA, eds. *Duane's Clinical Ophthalmology*. Philadelphia: Lippincott; 1998.

Thomas JV, Belcher CD III, Simmons RJ, eds. *Glaucoma Surgery*. St Louis: Mosby; 1992.

Zimmerman TJ, Kooner KS, Sharir M, Fechtner RD. *Textbook of Ocular Pharmacology*. Philadelphia: Lippincott; 1997.

# RELATED ACADEMY MATERIALS

## Focal Points: Clinical Modules for Ophthalmologists

Balyeat HD. Cataract surgery in the glaucoma patient, part 1: a cataract surgeon's perspective (Module 3, 1998).

Beck AD, Lynch MG. Pediatric glaucoma (Module 5, 1997).

Camras CB. Diagnosis and management of complications of glaucoma filtering surgery (Module 3, 1994).

Drake MV. A primer on automated perimetry (Module 8, 1993).

Gross RL. Cyclodestructive procedures for glaucoma (Module 4, 1992).

Heuer D, Lloyd MA. Management of glaucomas with poor surgical prognoses (Module 1, 1995).

Jampel HD. Normal (low) tension glaucoma (Module 12, 1991).

Lieberman MF. Glaucoma and automated perimetry (Module 9, 1993).

Liebmann JM. Pigmentary glaucoma: new insights (Module 2, 1998).

Lundy DC. Ciliary block glaucoma (Module 3, 1999).

Lynch MC, Brown RH. Systemic side effects of glaucoma therapy (Module 4, 1990).

McGrath DJ, Ferguson JG Jr., Sanborn GE. Neovascular glaucoma (Module 7, 1997).

Mikelberg FS. Normal-tension glaucoma: the next generation of glaucoma management (Module 12, 2000).

Mitrev PV, Schuman JS. Lasers in glaucoma management (Module 9, 2001).

Moster MR, Azuara-Blanco A. Techniques of glaucoma filtration surgery (Module 6, 2000).

Panek WC. Role of laser treatment in glaucoma (Module 1, 1993).

Ritch R. Exfoliation syndrome (Module 9, 1994).

Rockwood EJ. Medical treatment of open-angle glaucoma (Module 10, 1993).

Samples JR. Management of glaucoma secondary to uveitis (Module 5, 1995).

Schwartz B. Optic disc evaluation in glaucoma (Module 12, 1990).

Serle JB, Podos SM. New therapeutic options for the treatment of glaucoma (Module 5, 1999).

Skuta GL. Cataract surgery in the glaucoma patient, part 2: a glaucoma surgeon's perspective (Module 4, 1998).

# Publications

Alward WA. *Color Atlas of Gonioscopy* (2000).

Lane SS, Skuta GL, eds. *ProVision: Preferred Responses in Ophthalmology.* Series 3 (Self-Assessment Program, 1999).

Netland PA, Allen RC, eds. *Glaucoma Medical Therapy: Principles and Management* (Ophthalmology Monograph 13, 1999).

Skuta GL, ed. *ProVision: Preferred Responses in Ophthalmology.* Series 2 (Self-Assessment Program, 1996).

Walsh TJ, ed. *Visual Fields: Examination and Interpretation.* 2nd ed. (Ophthalmology Monograph 3, 1996).

Weinreb RN, Mills RP, eds. *Glaucoma Surgery: Principles and Techniques.* 2nd ed. (Ophthalmology Monograph 4, 1998).

Wilson FM II, ed. *Practical Ophthalmology: A Manual for Beginning Residents* (1996).

# Slide-Script

Coleman A. *Glaucoma: Diagnosis and Management* (Eye Care Skills for the Primary Care Physician Series, 1999).

# Multimedia

*Eye Care Skills on CD-ROM* (all seven titles from the Eye Care Skills for the Primary Care Physician Series) (2001).

*ProVision Interactive: Clinical Case Studies.* (Volume 2: Retina and Glaucoma on CD-ROM, 1997).

Sherwood MB, Brandt JD, Choplin NT, et al. *LEO Clinical Update Course on Glaucoma* (CD-ROM, 2001).

# Continuing Ophthalmic Video Education

Carassa RG, Bettin P, Brancato R. *Viscocanalostomy;* and Negri-Aranguren I, Acosta J. *Viscocanalostomy: The New Alternative in Glaucoma Surgery?* (1999).

Lewis RA. *Goldmann Applanation Tonometry* (1988).

Morris RE, Witherspoon CD, Kuhn F, et al. *Forceps Removal of the Retinal Internal Limiting Membrane in Surgery for Macular Hole and Macular Pucker;* John T. *New Surgical Technique for the Management of Exposed Ahmed Valve Tube;* and John T. *Penetrating Keratoplasty, Ahmed Valve, and Pericardial Graft* (2000).

Ramanathan US, Choi JTL, Kumar V, et al. *Lamellar Scleral Patch Graft for the Repair of Leaking Trabeculectomy Bleb with Full-Thickness Scleral Deficits;* Prasad KK, Garudadri CS, Mandal AK, et al. *Gonioscopy: Learn and Teach;* Cohn HC. *The Evolution of Glaucoma Filtering Surgery* (2001).

# Preferred Practice Patterns

Preferred Practice Patterns Committee, Glaucoma Panel. *Primary Open-Angle Glaucoma Suspect* (2000).

Preferred Practice Patterns Committee, Glaucoma Panel. *Primary Angle Closure* (2000).

Preferred Practice Patterns Committee, Glaucoma Panel. *Primary Open-Angle Glaucoma* (2000).

# Ophthalmic Technology Assessments

Ophthalmic Technology Assessment Committee. *Automated Perimetry* (1995).

Ophthalmic Technology Assessment Committee. *Cyclophotocoagulation* (2002).

Ophthalmic Technology Assessment Committee. *Laser Peripheral Iridotomy for Pupillary-Block Glaucoma* (1994).

Ophthalmic Technology Assessment Committee. *Laser Trabeculoplasty for Primary Open-Angle Glaucoma* (1996).

Ophthalmic Technology Assessment Committee. *Nonpenetrating Glaucoma Surgery* (2001).

Ophthalmic Technology Assessment Committee. *Optic Nerve Head and Retinal Nerve Fiber Layer Analysis* (1999).

# Complementary Therapy Assessments

Complementary Therapy Task Force. *Marijuana in the Treatment of Glaucoma* (2000).

# LEO Clinical Topic Updates Online

Brandt JD. *Glaucoma* (2000).

---

To order any of these materials, please call the Academy's Customer Service number at (415) 561-8540.

# CREDIT REPORTING FORM

## BASIC AND CLINICAL SCIENCE COURSE
### Section 10
## 2002–2003

*CME Accreditation*

The American Academy of Ophthalmology is accredited by the Accreditation Council for Continuing Medical Education to provide continuing medical education for physicians.

The American Academy of Ophthalmology designates this educational activity for a maximum of 30 hours in category 1 credit toward the AMA Physician's Recognition Award. Each physician should claim only those hours of credit that he/she has actually spent in the activity.

If you wish to claim continuing medical education credit for your study of this section, you must send this page and the following 3 pages (by mail or FAX) to the Academy office. Please make sure to:

1. Fill in and sign the statement below.
2. Write your answers to the questions on the back of this form.
3. Complete the study questions and mark your answers on the Section Completion Form.
4. Complete the Section Evaluation.

**Important: These completed forms must be received at the Academy within 3 years of purchase.**

I hereby certify that I have spent _____ (up to 30) hours of study on the curriculum of this section and that I have completed the study questions. (The Academy, *upon request,* will send you a verification of your Academy credits earned within the last 3 years.)

☐ *Please send credit verification now.*

Signature _____
                                                                    Date

Name: _____

Address: _____

City and State: _____ Zip: _____

Telephone: (_____) _____     *Academy Member ID# _____
                   area code

\* *Your ID number is located following your name on any Academy mailing label and on your Monthly Statement of Account.*

*Please return completed form to:*     **American Academy of Ophthalmology**
                                        **P.O. Box 7424**
                                        **San Francisco, CA 94120-7424**
                                        **ATTN: Clinical Education Division**

# READER'S RESPONSES

1. Please list several ways in which your study of this section will affect your practice.

2. How can we improve this section to better meet your continuing educational needs?

3. (OPTIONAL) Please list any topics you would like to see covered in other Academy clinical education products.

**BASIC AND CLINICAL SCIENCE COURSE**
ANSWER SHEET FOR SECTION 10

| Question | Answer | Question | Answer |
|---|---|---|---|
| 1 | a  b  c  d | 18 | a  b  c  d |
| 2 | a  b  c  d  e | 19 | a  b  c  d |
| 3 | a  b  c  d | 20 | a  b  c  d  e |
| 4 | a  b  c  d  e | 21 | a  b  c  d  e |
| 5 | a  b  c  d  e | 22 | a  b  c  d  e |
| 6 | a  b  c  d | 23 | a  b  c  d  e |
| 7 | a  b  c  d | 24 | a  b  c  d  e |
| 8 | a  b  c  d  e | 25 | a  b  c  d  e |
| 9 | a  b  c  d | 26 | a  b  c  d  e |
| 10 | a  b  c  d  e | 27 | a  b  c  d  e |
| 11 | a  b  c  d  e | 28 | a  b  c  d |
| 12 | a  b  c  d | 29 | a  b  c  d |
| 13 | a  b  c  d  e | 30 | a  b  c  d |
| 14 | a  b  c  d  e | 31 | a  b  c  d |
| 15 | a  b  c  d | 32 | a  b  c  d |
| 16 | a  b  c  d | 33 | a  b  c  d  e |
| 17 | a  b  c  d  e | 34 | a  b  c  d  e |

Please complete the Section Evaluation on the back of this page.

# SECTION EVALUATION

Please indicate your response to the statements listed below by placing the appropriate number to the left of each statement.

1 =agree strongly
2 =agree
3 =no opinion
4 =disagree
5 =strongly disagree

\_\_\_\_\_ This section meets its stated objectives.

\_\_\_\_\_ This section helped me keep current on this topic.

\_\_\_\_\_ I will apply knowledge gained from this section to my practice.

\_\_\_\_\_ This section covers topics in sufficient depth and detail.

\_\_\_\_\_ This section's illustrations are of sufficient number and quality.

\_\_\_\_\_ The references included in the text provide an appropriate amount of additional reading.

\_\_\_\_\_ The study questions at the end of the book are useful.

# STUDY QUESTIONS

# STUDY QUESTIONS

The following multiple-choice questions are designed to be used after your course of study with this book. Record your responses on the answer sheet (the Section Completion Form) by circling the appropriate letter. For the most effective use of this exercise, *complete the entire test* before consulting the answers.

Although a concerted effort has been made to avoid ambiguity and redundancy in these questions, the authors recognize that differences of opinion may occur regarding the "best" answer. The discussions are provided to demonstrate the rationale used to derive the answer. They may also be helpful in confirming that your approach to the problem was correct or, if necessary, in fixing the principle in your memory. Where relevant, additional textbook and journal references are given.

1. In the physiology of aqueous humor formation, the process that is energy-dependent and independent of the intraocular pressure is

    a. Ultrafiltration
    b. Active transport
    c. Simple diffusion
    d. Bulk flow

2. The prevalence of glaucoma is

    a. Equal in blacks and whites
    b. Two times more common in whites than in blacks
    c. Eight to ten times more common in whites than in blacks
    d. Three to six times higher in blacks than in whites
    e. Two times higher in blacks than in whites

3. The blood–aqueous barrier function of the ciliary body is

    a. Related to tight junctions within the pigmented epithelium as a result of cellular membrane permeability restrictions
    b. Related to tight junctions between the apexes of nonpigmented epithelial cells
    c. Related to the integrity and lack of permeability of the vascular elements within the ciliary body
    d. The reason the aqueous and blood concentration of ascorbate are the same

4. The following statements about static threshold perimetry are all true *except:*

    a. It allows high-quality perimetry to be performed by perimetrists who have not undergone extensive training.
    b. It is easy for the patient.
    c. The results depend on the size and luminance of the stimulus.
    d. The data can be summarized and analyzed using statistical programs.
    e. The results need to be interpreted in light of the patient's overall clinical picture.

5. The drawing shows a Zeiss gonioprism on the patient's right eye. The clock hour of *angle* that corresponds to the X is

   a.   11:00
   b.   1:00
   c.   4:00
   d.   7:00
   e.   6:00

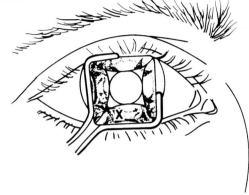

6. The following statements all characterize normal vessels in the angle *except:*

   a.   They frequently branch out over the trabecular meshwork in the inter-palpebral space.
   b.   They are radial.
   c.   They may run circumferentially around the periphery and be visible in only part of the angle.
   d.   They originate from the iris, ciliary body, and anterior ciliary arteries.

7. Elevated IOP (≥22 mm Hg) is

   a.   Commonly caused by alcohol consumption, particularly in individuals who are not regular consumers of alcohol
   b.   Caused in part by defective autoregulation of the peripapillary capillaries
   c.   A risk factor for the development of glaucoma
   d.   All of the above

8. The Goldmann applanation tonometer

   a.   Is of little value in individuals with >5 D of corneal astigmatism
   b.   Is not affected by alteration in scleral rigidity or by corneal thickness
   c.   Displaces approximately 50 μl of fluid from the anterior chamber
   d.   Is the most valid and reliable of currently available applanation devices
   e.   All of the above

9. All of the following statements regarding Goldmann applanation tonometry are true *except:*

   a.   The diameter of the applanated area is 3.06 mm.
   b.   The tear film creates surface tension that increases the force of applanation.
   c.   The cornea tends to resist deformation, which tends to balance out the surface tension effect of the tear film.
   d.   The IOP tends to be overestimated in eyes with low scleral rigidity.

10. Which of the following visual field defects is most characteristic of glaucoma?

    a.   Bitemporal hemianopia
    b.   Paracentral scotoma
    c.   Central scotoma
    d.   Superior quadrant anopia
    e.   Inferior quadrant anopia

11. Each of the following conditions may produce nerve fiber bundle visual field defects similar to those seen in glaucoma *except:*

    a.   Chronic papilledema
    b.   Optic disc drusen
    c.   AION
    d.   Occipital infarction
    e.   Branch retinal artery occlusion

12. Glaucoma with statistically normal intraocular pressure

    a.   Is relatively rare
    b.   Should be routinely investigated with CT scans for possibility of tumor
    c.   Can be differentiated from glaucoma with elevated IOP by visual fields and optic nerve characteristics
    d.   None of the above

13. The following are histologic changes in glaucoma *except:*

    a.   Posterior bowing of the lamina cribrosa
    b.   Thinning of the retinal nerve fiber layer
    c.   Loss of the outer nuclear layer of the retina
    d.   Loss of ganglion cells in the retina
    e.   Peripapillary atrophy of the choroid

14. Secondary angle closure with pupillary block is the usual mechanism for glaucoma in each of the following *except:*

    a.   An intumescent lens
    b.   Iris neovascularization
    c.   Microspherophakia
    d.   Uveitis
    e.   Ectopia lentis

15. The iridocorneal endothelial (ICE) syndromes include all of the following *except:*

    a.   Chandler syndrome
    b.   Axenfeld-Rieger syndrome
    c.   Iris nevus syndrome
    d.   Essential iris atrophy

16. A patient with nanophthalmos presents with angle-closure glaucoma. Your attempts at laser peripheral iridectomy are unsuccessful. Your next procedure should be

    a. Trabeculectomy
    b. Combined phacoemulsification and cataract extraction
    c. Surgical peripheral iridectomy
    d. Argon laser gonioplasty or iridoplasty

17. Ciliary block glaucoma, or malignant glaucoma, is associated with all of the following *except:*

    a. Responds to aqueous suppressant and hyperosmotic medical management in approximately 50% of cases
    b. Secondary posterior misdirection of aqueous into the vitreous cavity occurs
    c. Occurs only after incisional surgery and never following laser treatment
    d. Occurs most commonly in eyes with a history of angle-closure glaucoma
    e. May occur in aphakic or pseudophakic eyes

18. Which of the following causes of developmental glaucoma does *not* involve trabeculodysgenesis as a part of its pathophysiology?

    a. Sturge-Weber
    b. Homocystinuria
    c. Aniridia
    d. Peters anomaly

19. Which of the following statements about primary congenital glaucoma is *false?*

    a. 80% of cases are diagnosed by 1 year of age.
    b. 70%–75% of cases are bilateral.
    c. Most inherited cases are autosomal dominant.
    d. 65% of patients are male.

20. Which of the following beta blockers demonstrates the relative selectivity in the manner described?

    a. Betaxolol: relatively selective for $beta_2$ receptors
    b. Timolol: relatively selective for $beta_1$ receptors
    c. Levobunolol: relatively selective for $beta_2$ receptors
    d. Betaxolol: relatively selective for $beta_1$ receptors
    e. Levobunolol: relatively selective for $beta_1$ receptors

21. The following statements concerning pilocarpine are true *except:*

    a. By relaxing tension on the zonular fibers, it may cause narrowing of the anterior chamber.
    b. It is a direct cholinergic agonist.
    c. It reduces IOP by increasing aqueous outflow.
    d. It inhibits acetylcholinesterase.
    e. It is relatively contraindicated in the treatment of uveitic glaucoma.

22. The following statements regarding the topical carbonic anhydrase inhibitor dorzolamide are true *except:*

    a.  It lowers IOP by decreasing aqueous production.
    b.  Difficulties with ocular penetration prolonged the development of this compound.
    c.  It has the potential for side effects similar to those of systemic carbonic anhydrase inhibitors, though less frequent.
    d.  It has been shown to be clinically effective for once-daily administration.
    e.  It may cause Stevens-Johnson syndrome.

23. The agent most likely to be associated with follicular conjunctivitis is

    a.  Carbachol
    b.  Betaxolol
    c.  Brimonidine
    d.  Dorzolamide
    e.  Timolol

24. When performing argon laser trabeculoplasty, the most appropriate laser settings are

    a.  200-µm spot size, 0.2-sec duration, 600-mW power
    b.  50-µm spot size, 0.1-sec duration, 800-mW power
    c.  100-µm spot size, 0.5-sec duration, 1500-mW power
    d.  50-µm spot size, 0.1-sec duration, 1500-mW power
    e.  100-µm spot size, 0.1-sec duration, 800-mW power

25. The following early complications have been associated with filtering surgery *except:*

    a.  Corneal vascularization
    b.  Endophthalmitis
    c.  Hypotony maculopathy
    d.  Cystoid macular edema
    e.  Loss of vision

26. Indications for combined cataract and filtering surgery include all of the following *except:*

    a.  Uncontrolled glaucoma when vision is significantly impaired by cataract
    b.  Visually significant cataract in a glaucoma patient with advanced field loss
    c.  Visually significant glaucoma in a patient poorly tolerant of medical therapy
    d.  Visually significant cataract in a patient requiring multiple medications to control IOP
    e.  Visually significant cataract and very high IOP from acute pupillary block

27. Glaucoma drainage device implantation may be indicated when IOP is uncontrolled in all of the following *except:*

    a.   Failed trabeculectomy with antifibrotics
    b.   Blind painful eye with neovascular glaucoma
    c.   Active uveitis
    d.   Inadequate limbal conjunctiva
    e.   Following scleral buckle and vitrectomy

28. The secondary angle-closure glaucoma in which the PAS extend anterior to Schwalbe's line is

    a.   Axenfeld-Rieger syndrome
    b.   Neovascular glaucoma
    c.   ICE syndrome
    d.   Fuchs heterochromic iridocyclitis

29. The form of primary angle-closure glaucoma that does *not* have pupillary block as its only mechanism for angle closure is

    a.   Aniridia
    b.   Acute angle-closure glaucoma
    c.   Subacute angle-closure glaucoma
    d.   Plateau iris

30. The condition in which iris neovascularization is *not* associated with peripheral anterior synechiae and secondary angle closure is

    a.   Fuchs heterochromic iridocyclitis
    b.   Ocular ischemic syndrome
    c.   Central retinal vein occlusion
    d.   Chronic retinal detachment

31. The prevalence of primary open-angle glaucoma is higher in all of the following populations *except:*

    a.   Blacks versus whites
    b.   Patients with elevated intraocular pressure
    c.   Seventy-year-old women versus 80-year-old men
    d.   Patients with a primary relative with known primary open-angle glaucoma

32. An 80-year-old white male presents with poor vision in his right eye with sudden onset of pain and conjunctival hyperemia. The examination reveals an IOP of 45 with a prominent cell and flare reaction without keratic precipitates, a dense cataract, and an open anterior chamber angle. The most likely diagnosis is

    a.   Phacolytic glaucoma
    b.   Phacoanaphylaxis
    c.   ICE syndrome
    d.   Fuchs heterochromic iridocyclitis

33. The following ocular side effects have all been associated with the use of latanoprost *except:*

    a.  Hypertrichosis
    b.  Increased iris pigmentation
    c.  Cystoid macular edema
    d.  Decreased uveoscleral outflow
    e.  Periocular pigmentation

34. The following are all associated with the use of brimonidine *except:*

    a.  Increased uveoscleral outflow
    b.  Nonselective alpha agonist
    c.  Follicular conjunctivitis
    d.  Additivity to beta blocker
    e.  IOP lowering equivalent to timolol

# ANSWERS

1. Answer—b. Active transport consumes energy and moves substances against an electrochemical gradient. This process is pressure-independent.

2. Answer—d. The prevalence of glaucoma in the black population is estimated to be three to six times higher than in the white population. In addition, the disease tends to occur at an earlier age in the black population and more commonly results in blindness.

3. Answer—b. The tight junctional barrier between the apexes of nonpigmented epithelial cells presents a selective barrier, which allows diffusion of water and small molecules into the posterior chamber and therefore makes up the blood–aqueous barrier.

4. Answer—b. Most patients find static threshold perimetry fatiguing and unpleasant. It requires an extended period of concentration. Nevertheless, it is extremely valuable.

5. Answer—a. The Zeiss gonioprism mirrors are flat and do not reverse left for right. The superior angle is seen in the inferior mirror, but the nasal and temporal orientation is not changed.

6. Answer—a. Vessels that branch out over the trabecular meshwork are not normal. The two conditions most commonly associated with vessels branching over the trabecular meshwork are diabetes with proliferative retinopathy and central retinal vein occlusion.

7. Answer—c. Alcohol transiently decreases IOP, and the peripapillary capillaries have no known effect on IOP. The possibility of capillary autoregulation is an area of current research.

8. Answer—d. Goldmann applanation tonometry is valid in patients with high corneal astigmatism, but the technique must be modified. Alterations in scleral rigidity and corneal thickness do affect readings. Only 0.5 µl of fluid is displaced by Goldmann tonometry.

9. Answer—d. The IOP in eyes with low scleral rigidity may be underestimated with applanation tonometry, although this effect is more pronounced when techniques of indentation tonometry are used.

10. Answer—b. Choices a, d, and e are neurologic defects. A central scotoma is not typical of glaucoma.

11. Answer—d. All of the choices except occipital infarction may produce nerve fiber bundle defects, which can mimic the visual field loss seen in glaucoma. Occipital infarction would typically produce a homonymous hemianopia.

12. Answer—c. The temporal and inferotemporal neuroretinal rim are most affected early in normal-tension glaucoma, although other patterns of disc damage may also be observed.

13. Answer—c. Loss of the outer nuclear layer is not observed in glaucoma. Glaucoma results in loss of ganglion cells and their axons, which make up the retinal nerve fiber layer.

14. Answers—b. All of these conditions are associated with pupillary block except iris neovascularization, which usually causes glaucoma initially by an open-angle mechanism and later by peripheral anterior synechiae.

15. Answer—b. Iris nevus syndrome, Chandler syndrome, and essential iris atrophy are the three characteristic syndromes that relate to the spectrum of findings that may be seen in the iridocorneal endothelial syndromes. Axenfeld-Rieger syndrome is a disorder of the iris stroma that may have other associated ocular and systemic abnormalities.

16. Answer—d. Intraocular surgery in nanophthalmic eyes is fraught with complications, including choroidal effusions and nonrhegmatogenous retinal detachment. Argon laser gonioplasty should be attempted if peripheral iridectomy is unsuccessful.

17. Answer—c. Ciliary block, or malignant, glaucoma is characterized by a shallow anterior chamber with elevated IOP as a result of posterior misdirection of aqueous. It occurs most commonly following intraocular surgery in eyes with a history of angle-closure glaucoma but may also follow laser iridectomy or other procedures. It has been reported in aphakic and pseudophakic eyes as well as phakic eyes.

18. Answer—b. Trabeculodysgenesis is probably the most common pathophysiologic mechanism behind the entire category of developmental glaucomas. It has never been reported in homocystinuria.

19. Answer—c. Most of the inherited cases (only 10% of all cases) are autosomal recessive.

20. Answer—d. Because of its relative beta$_1$ selectivity, betaxolol has fewer pulmonary side effects. Timolol and levobunolol are nonselective beta blockers.

21. Answer—d. An indirect cholinergic agonist would inhibit cholinesterase. Pilocarpine is a direct-acting cholinergic agonist.

22. Answer—d. Dorzolamide has been approved for three-times-daily dosing.

23. Answer—c. Any topical agent can potentially produce either allergic or toxic surface reaction. However, brimonidine is the agent most likely to be associated with follicular conjunctivitis.

24. Answer—b. A 50-μm spot size of 0.1-second duration is preferred for laser trabeculoplasty. Initial power settings are usually between 600 and 800 mW and then adjusted as necessary to obtain a blanch or occasional small bubble formation in the meshwork.

25. Answer—a. Endophthalmitis, hypotony, maculopathy, cystoid macular edema, and loss of vision are among the early complications associated with filtering surgery.

26. Answer—e. Pupillary block should be managed with medical reduction of IOP and iridectomy. Cataract surgery can be performed when the eye is quiet. Filtering surgery may be unnecessary.

27. Answer—b. Incisional surgery should rarely, if ever, be performed on a blind eye.

28. Answer—c. ICE syndrome has an abnormal corneal endothelium that allows for the PAS to extend anterior to Schwalbe's line. Neovascular glaucoma and Fuchs heterochromic iridocyclitis have a normal corneal endothelium. In Axenfeld-Rieger syndrome, Schwalbe's line is displaced anteriorly; however, the PAS are limited to this anterior displacement.

29. Answer—d. Plateau iris is the only form of primary angle closure that is not totally caused by a pupillary-block mechanism. Acute and subacute angle-closure glaucoma are primary angle-closure glaucomas in which the cause of the angle closure is secondary to pupillary block. Aniridia is a form of secondary angle closure.

30. Answer—a. Fine neovascularization of the iris and anterior chamber angle occurs in Fuchs heterochromic iridocyclitis, but it is not associated with angle closure and PAS formation. The other three conditions can cause iris neovascularization associated with PAS and secondary angle-closure glaucoma.

31. Answer—c. The major risk factors for primary open-angle glaucoma are increased intraocular pressure, race, increasing age, and known family history. The prevalence of primary open-angle glaucoma is relatively equal between the sexes.

32. Answer—a. This is the classic presentation of a patient with phacolytic glaucoma. Without keratic precipitates, both phacoanaphylaxis and Fuchs heterochromic iridocyclitis are unlikely. Fuchs heterochromic iridocyclitis is associated with cataract formation, primarily posterior subcapsular cataracts, but it tends to present in a much younger patient. ICE syndrome occurs in younger patients and causes a secondary angle-closure glaucoma.

33. Answer—d. Latanoprost is associated with increased uveoscleral outflow. All of the other answers are known to occur.

34. Answer—b. Brimonidine is a selective alpha$_2$ agonist.

# INDEX

treatment of
  medical, 146
  surgical, 163–166, 164*i*
  tumors causing, 115
Angle recession, posttraumatic, 36–37,
  38*i*, 93–94, 93*i*
  glaucoma and, 36, 93–94
Aniridia
  gene for, 13*t*
  glaucoma associated with, 122
Anterior chamber
  blunt trauma to, 37, 38*i*, 92–96
  evaluation of in glaucoma, 28–29, 28*t*
  flat
    angle-closure glaucoma and,
      104–105, 121
    re-formation (deepening) surgery and,
      160, 166
Anterior chamber angle
  blood vessels in, 35–36, 36*i*
  in exfoliation syndrome, 82, 83*i*
  gonioscopy of, in glaucoma, 30, 30*i*, 31*i*
  in infants/children, 124
  measurement of width of, 34
  narrow, angle-closure glaucoma and,
    104–105
  neovascularization of, angle-closure
    glaucoma and, 36, 110–113, 110*t*,
    111*i*, 112*i*, 168
  traumatic recession of, 36–37, 38*i*,
    93–94, 93*i*
  glaucoma and, 36, 93–94
Anterior chamber tube shunt to an
  encircling band (ACTSEB), 166–167
Anterior segment
  in exfoliation syndrome, 82–83
  trauma to, 92–98
    blunt, 37, 38*i*, 92–96, 92*i*, 93*i*, 95*i*, 96*i*
    chemical, 93
    surgical, 97–98
Anterior synechiae
  in angle-closure glaucoma, 103, 110,
    112*i*, 115, 116*i*
    chamber deepening procedures
      and, 166
  gonioscopy in identification of, 32, 33*i*,
    36, 37*i*
  iris processes differentiated from, 36, 37*i*
Anticholinesterase agents, 134*t*, 139

Antifibrotic agents
  with filtering procedures, 153, 159
  glaucoma tube shunts and, 167
  for neovascular glaucoma, 113
  for normal-tension glaucoma, 81
Antiglaucoma agents, 131–144, 132–136*t*.
  *See also specific type*
  adrenergic agonists, 132–133*t*, 141–143
  beta blockers, 132*t*, 137–138
  carbonic anhydrase inhibitors, 135*t*,
    140–141
  combined medications, 136*t*, 143–144
  hyperosmotic, 136*t*, 144
  interrelationship between medical and
    surgical treatment and, 131
  parasympathomimetic (miotic) agents,
    134*t*, 138–139
  prostaglandin analogues, 136*t*, 143
  risk-benefit assessment and, 130–131
Aphakic glaucoma, 108–109
Applanation tonometer (applanation
  tonometry), 20–23, 21*i*, 22*i*
  infection control and, 23–24
  portable devices for, 23–24
Apraclonidine, 133*t*, 142, 143
Aqueous humor, 14
  formation of, 14–16
    rate of, 16
    suppression of, 15–16
  intraocular pressure and, 14–24
  outflow of, 16–18
    tonography for measurement of, 18
    trabecular, 16–17, 17*i*
    uveoscleral, 17–18
Aqueous misdirection (malignant/ciliary
  block glaucoma; posterior aqueous
  diversion syndrome), 117
Arcuate scotoma, in glaucoma, 53*i*
Argon laser therapy
  for ciliary ablation in glaucoma, 170
  iridectomy, for angle-closure glaucoma,
    163, 164–165
  photocoagulation, for aqueous
    misdirection (ciliary block/
    malignant glaucoma), 117
  trabeculoplasty, for open-angle
    glaucoma, 149, 150*i*
Armaly-Drance screening perimetry, 69, 70*i*
Arteriovenous fistulae, glaucoma
  associated with, 26

Arthro-ophthalmopathy, hereditary
   progressive (Stickler syndrome),
   childhood glaucoma and, 128t
Artifacts, in visual field testing, 61–62,
   63–64i
Ash-leaf spot, 26
Automated perimetry, static, 50, 51, 58–69
   artifacts seen on, 61–62, 63i, 64i
   high false-negative rate in, 62
   high false-positive rate in, 62, 64i
   incorrect corrective lens used in, 61
   learning effect and, 65, 66i
Autoregulation, disturbances of in
   glaucoma, 40, 42, 76
Axenfeld-Rieger syndrome
   gene for, 13, 13t
   glaucoma associated with, 26, 28, 122
Azopt. See Brinzolamide

Background, as perimetry variable, 57
Baerveldt implant, 166, 166t, 167i
Beta-adrenergic antagonists. See
      Beta blockers
Beta blockers
   aqueous formation affected by, 15, 137
   for glaucoma, 132t, 137–138
      in children, 126
      in combined medication form, 137, 144
   side effects of, 132t, 137–138
Betagan. See Levobunolol
Betanorm. See Metipranolol, with
   pilocarpine
Betaxolol, 132t, 137
Betimol. See Timolol
Betoptic. See Betaxolol
Bimatoprost, 135t, 143
Biomicroscopy
   slit-lamp
      in glaucoma evaluation, 27–29, 30i
      for optic disc evaluation, 29, 43
   ultrasound
      in glaucoma, 70, 71i
      for plateau iris identification, 105, 105i
Blepharospasm, in congenital/infantile
   glaucoma, 124
Blindness, glaucoma causing, 10
Blood pressure
   intraocular pressure and, 76
   open-angle glaucoma and, 76
Blue/yellow perimetry, 50
Blunt trauma, anterior segment, glaucoma
   and, 37, 38i, 92–96, 92i, 93i, 95i, 96i

Bourneville syndrome (tuberous sclerosis),
   glaucoma associated with, 26
Brimonidine, 133t, 142–143
Brinzolamide, 135t, 140, 141
Broad thumb syndrome (Rubinstein-Taybi
   syndrome), childhood glaucoma
   and, 128t
Buphthalmos (megaloglobus), in childhood
   glaucoma, 122, 124

CAIs. See Carbonic anhydrase inhibitors
Calcium channel blockers, for
   normal-tension glaucoma, 81
Capsular block, 109
Capsulotomy, posterior, pupillary block
   after, 109
Carbachol, 134t, 138
Carbonic anhydrase, in aqueous humor
   formation, 14
Carbonic anhydrase inhibitors
   aqueous formation affected by,
      15–16, 140
   for glaucoma, 134–135t, 140–141
      in children, 126
   side effects of, 135t, 140–141
Cardiovascular disorders, primary open-
   angle glaucoma associated with, 76
Carteolol, 132t, 137
Cataract
   hypermature, lens protein leakage from,
      phacolytic glaucoma caused by,
      86–87, 87i
   perimetry results affected by, 65
Cataract surgery
   in angle-closure glaucoma, 166
   filtering surgery combined with,
      162–163
   flat anterior chamber after, angle-closure
      glaucoma and, 121
   lens particle glaucoma after, 87–88, 88i
   pupillary block after, 109
Central island of vision, in glaucoma, 51, 56i
Central retinal vein, occlusion of
   angle-closure glaucoma and, 120
   open-angle glaucoma and, 76
Cerebrohepatorenal syndrome (Zellweger
   syndrome), childhood glaucoma
   and, 128t
Chalcosis, open-angle glaucoma and, 93
Chamber angle, anterior. See Anterior
   chamber angle
Chamber deepening procedures, for angle-
   closure glaucoma, 166

Hemorrhages, splinter, in glaucoma, 44–45, 45*i*

Hereditary factors, in glaucoma, 12–13, 13*t*, 122

Hereditary progressive arthro-ophthalmopathy (Stickler syndrome), childhood glaucoma and, 128*t*

Heterochromia iridis, Fuchs. *See* Fuchs heterochromic iridocyclitis/uveitis

High-pass resolution perimetry, 50

Hruby lens, with slit lamp, for optic disc evaluation, 43

Humorsol. *See* Demecarium

Humphrey pattern standard deviation index, 61

Humphrey STATPAC 2 program, 61, 62*i*

Humphrey Visual Field Analyzer, 50

Hypermature cataract, lens protein leakage from, phacolytic glaucoma caused by, 86–87, 87*i*

Hyperopia, angle-closure glaucoma and, 12, 26

Hyperosmotic agents, 136*t*, 144

Hypertension
ocular, 76–77
systemic, open-angle glaucoma and, 76

Hypotensive lipids, 135*t*, 143

Hyphema, glaucoma and, 94–95, 95*i*

ICE. *See* Iridocorneal endothelial syndrome

Imbert-Fick principle, in tonometry, 20

Increased intraocular pressure. *See* Elevated intraocular pressure

Indentation gonioscopy (pressure/compression gonioscopy), 32, 33*i*

Indentation tonometry (Schiøtz tonometry), 23
infection control and, 24

Indirect ophthalmoscopy, for optic disc evaluation, 43

Infantile glaucoma, 122. *See also* Glaucoma, childhood

Inflammation (ocular)
secondary angle-closure glaucoma and, 115, 116*i*
secondary open-angle glaucoma and, 89–90, 90*i*

Intraocular lenses
anterior chamber, pupillary block and, 97–98, 97*i*, 109
glaucoma caused by, 97–98, 97*i*, 109

Intraocular pressure, 18–24
aqueous humor dynamics and, 14–24
digital pressure for estimation of, 23
distribution of in population, 18, 19*i*
diurnal variations in, 20
drugs for lowering, 131–144, 132–136*t*. *See also* Antiglaucoma agents
elevated. *See* Elevated intraocular pressure
episcleral venous pressure and, 18, 91
factors determining, 5, 5*i*, 19
in glaucoma suspect, 76–77
increased. *See* Elevated intraocular pressure
measurement of, 20–23, 21*i*, 22*i*. *See also* Tonometry
in infants, 124
normal range for, 5, 18, 19*i*
in primary open-angle glaucoma, 72, 73*t*, 74*t*
surgery for lowering, 166–171. *See also* Filtering procedures; Laser therapy

Intraocular tumors
angle-closure glaucoma caused by, 115
open-angle glaucoma caused by, 88–89

Iopidine. *See* Apraclonidine

Iridectomy
for angle-closure glaucoma, 102–103, 166
for aqueous misdirection (ciliary block/malignant glaucoma), 117
for ectopia lentis, 107–108
for elevated intraocular pressure in hyphema, 95
laser, for angle-closure glaucoma, 102–103, 163–165. *See also* Laser iridectomy
for pigmentary glaucoma, 85, 86*i*
for plateau iris, 106
in trabeculectomy, 157, 157*i*

Iridocorneal endothelial syndrome, glaucoma in, 113–115, 114*i*, 115*i*

Iridocyclitis
Fuchs heterochromic, 90, 90*i*
chamber angle vessels in, 36
glaucoma and, 90, 90*i*
secondary open-angle glaucoma and, 89

Iridodysgenesis, gene for, 13*t*

Iridoplasty, for plateau iris syndrome, 106, 106*i*, 165

Normal-tension glaucoma, 7*t*, 78–81
  classification of, 7*t*
  clinical features of, 78–79
  diagnostic evaluation of, 79–80
  differential diagnosis of, 79, 80*t*
  optic disc hemorrhages in, 44–45, 45*i*
  prognosis and therapy for, 81
Normal-Tension Glaucoma Study, 73*t*, 81

OCT. *See* Optical coherence tomography
Octopus loss variance index, 61
Ocudose. *See* Timolol
Ocular adnexa, in glaucoma evaluation,
  26–27
Ocular hypertension. *See* Hypertension,
  ocular
Ocular Hypertension Treatment Study, 74*t*,
  77, 130
Oculocerebrorenal syndrome (Lowe
  syndrome), childhood glaucoma
  and, 128*t*
Oculodentodigital dysplasia/syndrome
  (Meyer-Schwickerath and Weyers
  syndrome), childhood glaucoma
  and, 128*t*
Oculodermal melanocytosis (nevus of
  Ota), glaucoma associated with, 26
Oculomandibulofacial dyscephaly
  (Hallermann-Streiff syndrome),
  childhood glaucoma and, 128*t*
Ocupress. *See* Carteolol
Ocusert. *See* Pilocarpine
Open-angle glaucoma, 7*t*, 9*i*, 72–99. *See
  also* Glaucoma
  classification of, 6, 7*t*
  filtering procedures for, 151–163. *See
    also* Filtering procedures
  gene for, 13*t*
  incisional surgery for, 151–163. *See also*
    Filtering procedures
  juvenile, 7*t*, 122. *See also* Glaucoma,
    childhood
    gene for, 12, 13*t*
  laser therapy for, 148–151, 150*i*
  management of
    medical, 145–146. *See also
      specific agent*
    surgical, 148–163, 150*i*, 154–158*i*.
      *See also specific procedure*
  mechanisms of outflow obstruction in, 8*t*

posttraumatic angle recession and, 36,
  93–94
primary, 7*t*, 9*i*, 10–11, 72–76
  clinical features of, 72–74
  disorders associated with, 75–76
  epidemiology of, 10–11
  hereditary and genetic factors in,
    12–13, 13*t*
  intraocular pressure in, 72, 73*t*, 74*t*
  prevalence of, 11
  risk factors for, 11, 74
secondary, 7*t*, 81–99
  drug use and, 98–99
  episcleral venous pressure increases
    and, 91–92, 91*i*, 91*t*
  exfoliation syndrome (pseudo-
    exfoliation) and, 81–83, 82*i*, 83*i*
  intraocular tumors causing, 88–89
  lens-induced, 86–88, 86*t*, 87*i*, 88*i*
  ocular inflammation and, 89–90, 90*i*
  pigmentary, 83–85, 84*i*, 85*i*, 86*i*
  trauma causing
    accidental, 92–96, 92*i*, 93*i*, 95*i*, 96*i*
    surgical, 97–98, 97*i*, 98*t*
Ophthalmopathy, thyroid, glaucoma
  associated with, 26
Ophthalmoscopy, for optic nerve head
  evaluation, 43
  confocal scanning laser ophthalmoscope
    for, 47
Optic atrophy, glaucomatous, 45–46, 46*i*
Optic disc (optic nerve head)
  anatomy of, 39–42, 40*i*, 41*i*
  blood supply of, 40, 41*i*
    autoregulation disturbances in
      glaucoma and, 40, 42
  clinical evaluation of, 29, 43–48
    grading of, 48
  cupping of, 42, 43–44, 43*t*, 44*i*, 44*t*,
    45*i*, 48
    in infants/children, 42, 124–125
  divisions of, 39–40, 40*i*
  examination of, 29, 43
    in infants/children, 124–125
  in glaucoma, 39–48
    primary open-angle glaucoma, 72–74
    recording of findings and, 48
    theories of damage and, 42
  hemorrhage of in glaucoma, 44–45, 45*i*
  laminar layer of, 39–40, 41*i*

Rescula. *See* Isopropyl unoprosterone
Retinal detachment
    angle-closure glaucoma and, 109
    nonrhegmatogenous (secondary),
        angle-closure glaucoma and, 109
    surgery for, angle-closure glaucoma
        and, 119–120
Retinal disease, vascular, angle-closure
    glaucoma and, 120
Retinal nerve fiber layer. *See* Nerve
    fiber layer
Retinal nerve fibers, distribution of, 39, 40*i*
Retinal surgery, angle-closure glaucoma
    after, 119–120
Retinal vein occlusion, central
    angle-closure glaucoma and, 120
    open-angle glaucoma and, 76
Retinopathy of prematurity, angle-closure
    glaucoma and, 121
Retrolaminar layer, of optic nerve head, 42
Retrolental fibroplasia. *See* Retinopathy of
    prematurity
Rieger syndrome. *See also* Axenfeld-Rieger
    syndrome
    gene for, 13*t*
Risk factors, in primary open-angle
    glaucoma, 11
Rubeosis iridis (iris neovascularization), in
    angle-closure glaucoma, 110–113,
    110*t*, 111*i*, 112*i*
Rubinstein-Taybi syndrome (broad thumb
    syndrome), childhood glaucoma
    and, 128*t*

Sampoelesi's line, 82, 83*i*
Scanning laser ophthalmoscopy, confocal,
    in optic nerve head evaluation, 47
Scanning laser polarimetry, for retinal
    nerve fiber evaluation, 47
Schiøtz tonometry (indentation
    tonometry), 23
    aqueous outflow measurements using, 18
    infection control and, 24
Schlemm's canal, 14
    aqueous outflow through, 14, 16–17, 17*i*
    gonioscopic visualization of, 34
Schwalbe's line
    as angle landmark, 29*i*, 33–34
    in Axenfeld-Rieger syndrome, 28
Sclera, in glaucoma, 27

Scleral buckle, angle-closure glaucoma
    after, 119–120
Scleral flap, in trabeculectomy, 154, 156*i*
    closure of, 157, 158*i*, 159
Scleral spur, as angle landmark, 29*i*, 33–34
Sclerectomy, full-thickness, 161, 161*i*
Sclerostomy, in trabeculectomy, 157, 157*i*
Scotomata
    arcuate, in glaucoma, 53*i*
    definition of, 51
    paracentral, in glaucoma, 52*i*
Scottish Glaucoma Trial, 73*t*
Screening tests for glaucoma
    perimetry for, 60, 60*i*
        Armaly-Drance, 69, 70*i*
Secondary open-angle glaucoma. *See*
        Open-angle glaucoma, secondary
Seidel test, in flat anterior chamber, 121
Selective laser trabeculoplasty, 151
Senile sclerosis, in normal-tension
    glaucoma, 78
Sex (gender), angle-closure glaucoma
    prevalence affected by, 12
Shaffer system, for gonioscopic grading, 34
Sickle cell disease (sickle cell anemia),
        open-angle glaucoma and, 92, 94–95
Siderosis, open-angle glaucoma and, 93
SITA (Swedish Interactive Thresholding
        Algorithm) testing (perimetry), 58–59
Slit-lamp examination. *See* Biomicroscopy,
    slit-lamp
Spaeth gonioscopic grading system, 34, 35*i*
Splinter hemorrhages, in glaucoma,
        44–45, 45*i*
Static perimetry, 50–51
STATPAC 2 program (Humphrey), 61, 62*i*
Stickler syndrome (hereditary progressive
        arthro-ophthalmopathy), childhood
        glaucoma and, 128*t*
Stimulus, as perimetry variable, 57–58
Stromal ingrowth (fibrous downgrowth),
        angle-closure glaucoma and,
        118–119, 119*i*
Sturge-Weber syndrome (encephalofacial
        angiomatosis), increased episcleral
        pressure and, 26
Superior vena cava syndrome, glaucoma
        associated with, 26
Suprathreshold testing (perimetry), 51, 58
    for screening, 60

UGH syndrome. *See* Uveitis-glaucoma-hyphema (UGH) syndrome
Ultrafiltration, in aqueous humor formation, 15
Ultrasound biomicroscopy
  in glaucoma, 70, 71*i*
  for plateau iris identification, 105, 105*i*
Unoprosterone, isopropyl, 135*t*, 143
Uvea (uveal tract)
  cysts of, angle-closure glaucoma caused by, 115
  melanomas of, angle-closure glaucoma caused by, 115
Uveitis
  in angle-closure glaucoma, 115–116, 116*i*
  glaucoma tube shunts in setting of, 167
Uveitis-glaucoma-hyphema (UGH) syndrome, 97*i*, 98
Uveoscleral outflow, 17–18

Van Herick method, for anterior chamber measurement, 28
Vascular system, of anterior chamber angle, 35–36, 36*i*
VECP/VEP/VER. *See* Visually evoked cortical potential (visual evoked response)
Viruses, ocular infection/inflammation caused by, open-angle glaucoma and, 89
Viscocanalostomy, 171
Visual field, 48, 49*i*
  cloverleaf, 62, 63*i*
Visual field defects
  in glaucoma, 5, 51, 52–56*i*
    correlation of with optic disc, 65–69
    in primary open-angle glaucoma, 72–74

progression of, 65, 67*i*, 68*i*, 70
in normal-tension glaucoma, 79
Visual field indices for perimetry, 61
  corrected loss variance, 61
  corrected pattern standard deviation, 61
  in serial field interpretation, 65
Visual field testing. *See also* Perimetry
  in glaucoma, 48–70, 71*i*
Visual reaction time, perimetry affected by, 58
Visually evoked cortical potential (visual evoked response), in glaucoma identification, 50
Vitrectomy
  angle-closure glaucoma after, 120
  for aqueous misdirection (ciliary block/malignant glaucoma), 117
Vitreoretinal surgery, angle-closure glaucoma and, 120
von Recklinghausen disease (neurofibromatosis), glaucoma associated with, 26

Wavelength, background/stimulus, perimetry affected by, 57

Xalatan. *See* Latanoprost
Xanthogranuloma, juvenile, glaucoma associated with, 26

Zeiss lens, for gonioscopy, 32
Zellweger syndrome (cerebrohepatorenal syndrome), childhood glaucoma and, 128*t*
Zonular dehiscence, angle-closure glaucoma caused by, 106

# ILLUSTRATIONS

The authors submitted the following figures for this revision. (Illustrations that were reproduced from other sources or submitted by contributors not on the committee are credited in the captions.)

Louis Cantor, MD: Figs III-7, III-15

Robert D. Fechtner, MD: Figs VIII-2, VIII-3B, VIII-4C, VIII-5, VIII-6B and C, VIII-7B, VIII-8C

Steven T. Simmons, MD: Figs IV-2, IV-7, IV-9, IV-11, IV-13 through IV-16, IV-18, IV-19, V-4 through V-6, V-9, V-10, V-12 through V-21, V-24 through V-28

M. Roy Wilson, MD: Figs IV-6, V-3, VIII-10